Crime and Social Policy

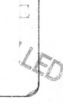

For Linda

Crime and Social Policy

The Police and Criminal Justice System

Mike Stephens
Senior Lecturer in Social Policy
Department of Social Sciences
Loughborough University

Gildredge Social Policy Series is published by:

The Gildredge Press Ltd
16 Gildredge Road
Eastbourne
East Sussex
BN21 4RL
United Kingdom

First Published 2000 by The Gildredge Press Ltd
Copyright © The Gildredge Press Ltd 2000

Cover Design: Clare Truscott
Cover Illustration: Alan McGowan/The Organisation
Typeset by Central Southern Typesetters, Eastbourne, East Sussex
Printed and Bound in Great Britain by Creative Print and Design Wales
ISBN 0–9533571–9–8

Contents

Tables

Appended Tables

Figures

Acknowledgements

During the writing of this book I have been fortunate to receive a great deal of support, encouragement and advice from several long-standing and very dear friends. My thanks go to Ian and Liz Aston, Allen Callaghan (who was more anxious than I that I finish the book on time!), Richard and Diane Cherry, Derek Edwards, Anne Lacey, Katie MacMillan, John and Marian Street and my brother Mark. I must also mention Norman Smith who was frequently a model of inscrutability but an inspiration nevertheless. Another valued friend of mine, David Russell, offered much helpful advice concerning the contents of Chapter 8. Naturally, any mistakes that remain in the text are my own. I was able in the Spring of 1998 to spend some time in America looking at policing and other aspects of the criminal justice system. In Chicago, the warmth and hospitality I received from Susan and James Witz and the great times I spent with their son, Jakey, will long live in my memory. In Madison, I owe a great debt to Sergeant Steven Cardarella who provided a thorough coverage of the Madison Police Department and the local mental health services. Not only is Steve a first-rate police officer, he and his family became my good friends.

Series introduction

Social policy in the United Kingdom has undergone major changes since the mid-1970s and particularly since the election of the Thatcher government in 1979. The post-war consensus is long gone and far-reaching changes have been made in every area of social policy. These changes, of principle and of practice, have been guided both by ideology and by the context of a post-industrial and increasingly globalized economy. The emergence of New Labour has added a new and still developing dimension of change.

The growing number of students of social policy, in higher education, on advanced level courses such as AS/A levels and GNVQs, and training for professional qualifications, have to make sense of this fast-changing scene, to consider the long-term effects, and to make their own judgements of the deep-rooted issues of value that are involved.

This new series of introductory textbooks is aimed specifically at these students. The books are not academic monographs but short, tightly-structured texts written with both the academic student and the trainee professional in mind. All the authors are currently involved in teaching and in policy development.

The books are designed to be aids to learning. Each book includes a brief history and background to its policy area, a review of current provision, and a discussion of future issues and possible developments. The books thus present students with a concise, clear and up-to-date summary of what they need to know and understand in each area of social policy.

Foreword

Skiing through the trees on Whistler Mountain in Canada was the last place in which I thought that the completion of this book would be on my mind. But Whistler employs so-called 'speed control' personnel who tour the slopes in their very long and bright yellow anoraks on the look out for those whom they consider to be skiing too quickly or out of control. If the piste police catch you, they can confiscate your lift pass and kick you off the slopes. In a way they are both judge and jury in their own cause and, while this kind of protection for other skiers seems perfectly valid at first glance, who is to say what is too fast, who is out of control? The whole purpose of the criminal justice system is not simply about detecting, processing and punishing wrong-doers, it is also about protecting those who are innocent and ensuring that justice is administered in an even-handed manner. This book is about the balance between the power of the state to punish criminals and the procedural safeguards that should apply to all citizens, even if they are the metaphorical equivalents of some crazy kid hurtling down the slope and about to crash.

Chapter 1 details the extent of crime in England and Wales, its problematic measurement, and how fear of crime may sometimes degenerate into a moral panic. Chapters 2 and 3 cover the police service, especially their powers of care and control and how these manifest themselves in different operational ways. Thus, included in the coverage are such topics as community policing and neighbourhood watch, the recruitment of women and ethnic minority officers, public order and paramilitary operations, stop and search, zero tolerance policing, and the nature of racism within the force. An overview of the criminal justice system is set out in Chapter 4 so that readers may understand not only the component organizational parts of that system, but also how they interact. Here the importance of due process and justice is emphasized and the work of each of the main agencies is summarized before I move on to a consideration of sentencing issues. Chapter 5 describes the nature of youth justice and the workings of the Youth Court, as well as indicating the scale of juvenile delinquency and the policy responses to it. The Magistrates' and Crown Courts are the focus of Chapter 6, in which I set out the role and workloads of these two forums and also delve into the topic of sentencing disparities and plea bargaining. There are also sections on race and justice, women and the courts and victims. Chapter 7 deals with prisons and penal policy and covers topics such as the organization and cost of the penal system, the composition of the prison population, the nature of the prison regime, the place of rehabilitative efforts, the impact of imprisonment, and the merits and otherwise of the 'prison works' philosophy. Community sentences such as probation, community service orders and electronic tagging are the main features of Chapter 8, as is a discussion of their worth within the available sentencing options. In the final chapter, the overall flaws within the criminal justice system are outlined, and recommendations are made to improve the quality of justice.

Throughout the text reference is made usually to the latest available figures and statistics at the time of writing, and every effort has been made to comment on the ideas and policies introduced by the Labour Government elected in May 1997.

Whistler, British Columbia

Crime and criminal justice in context

1

Outline

■ Many people are rightfully fearful of becoming victims of crime.

■ Among those most at risk are poorer people living in inner-city areas and run-down estates.

■ Many others, influenced by exaggerated media coverage of crime (especially of the violent kind), overestimate their chances of being victimized.

■ Most people have a poor factual knowledge of the true extent of crime.

CRIME AND SOCIETY

Crime, like poverty, is always with us. Indeed, the two are interrelated. Of course, it is individuals who commit crime, but there are societal patterns of crime that we must also take into account. The link between crime and poverty may be expressed in a number of ways, but one of the most revealing is the manner in which, after a suitable time-lag, certain kinds of crimes either increase or decrease following a change in the fortunes of the economy. The Home Office's Director of Research, Christopher Nuttall, has argued that 'the largest single determinant of the crime rate is the state of the economy' (*The Independent*, 18 September 1998, p. 13). Thus, when the economy is doing badly, there are more people out of work, and poverty is on the increase, property crimes, such as burglary and theft, tend to increase. When the economy is doing well and there are more people in work who have more money to spend, there is an increase in crimes of violence – largely as a result of more young men being able to go out more regularly, drink more alcohol, and more frequently become involved in various kinds of altercations.

Another link between crime and poverty can be found in the fact that 'the most crime-ridden communities tend also to be the poorest' (Wilson and Ashton 1998, p. 8). Moreover, both the official police-recorded statistics and the British Crime Survey showed that crime rates were much higher in lower income, urban communities whose inhabitants were also likely to become repeated victims (James and Raine 1998, p. 7).

Wealthier areas are not, however, immune to crime or to the fear of crime, since middle-class suburbs are frequently the target for burglaries. Fear of crime may also have devastating effects on people's lifestyles, with some individuals choosing to lock themselves into homes that have become mini-fortresses, and avoiding certain areas altogether – or deciding not to go out at night. In addition, crime is a costly business – and not just in terms of the financial and psychological costs that victims may incur. In 1994, crime was estimated to have cost £24.5 billion per year (Davies *et al.* 1998, p. 67).

THE PROBLEMATIC NATURE OF CRIME

Crime is not as straightforward as one might think; nor is it always as bad as media coverage might suggest. Previously many kinds of activities were illegal and severely punished. What is officially classified as a crime is not a fixed phenomenon; rather it evolves – sometimes indirectly according to public demands and the lobbying of interest groups, or directly according to the will of Parliament. For instance, not so many years ago everyone could drive their motorbikes legally without a crash helmet, whereas today it is illegal and clearly accepted as such by almost everyone, (including Hell's Angels). What is or isn't legally defined as a crime may alter over time according to different social and political circumstances. This not only makes it more difficult to define the exact nature of crime, it also creates difficulties in measuring how much crime has occurred – especially if the measurements span a lengthy period of time and one is trying to make comparisons. Despite these difficulties, England and Wales currently have two main ways of measuring crime, each with their own further problems. They are the annual official statistics of crime recorded by the police, and the biennial British Crime Survey. The Home Secretary, Jack Straw, indicated in 1997 that in future a more robust measuring system would be introduced to provide a more accurate picture of the extent of crime, which (on paper) will probably result in a significant increase in the recorded figures. Given the sensitivity surrounding crime figures in this country and the tendency to turn the issue into a moral panic, it will be most interesting to see how the media and politicians react to any such increase.

Measures of crime

(See the Appendix pp 132–135 for recent crime statistics)

The official crime figures recorded by the police contain a number of flaws. Clearly, many crimes go unrecorded because victims feel that the loss is too trivial to investigate, or that the police are powerless to help. On the other hand, the reporting of crime may significantly increase following a concerted advertising campaign, (for instance, to clamp down on burglary), and a similar increase in reporting may occur where the public hold 'new for old' insurance policies that encourage people to report thefts. In neither case will the real rate of crime have necessarily increased, but the reporting of it certainly will have (Wilson and Ashton 1998, p. 3). People may report crimes to the police, but for a variety of reasons the police may not record them as crimes and, therefore, they cannot appear in the official statistics. A 'no-crime' may be recorded by the police if the offence is trivial and the chances of solving it are not good. Moreover, recording practices differ considerably between police forces – as do their respective clear-up rates. Racially motivated crimes may now be separately classified, but the rigour with which police forces accurately record such offences varies greatly and, accordingly, the number of officially recorded crimes with a racial element is likely to be seriously underestimated. Finally, crimes involving a number of victims are often recorded as one crime instead of several – a practice the government intends to discontinue.

As a result of these kinds of difficulties with official statistics, the British Crime Survey (BCS) was first conducted in 1982 by the Home Office as a different approach to the measurement of crime. Essentially, the BCS is a random sample of almost 15,000 people aged 16 and over. Respondents are asked about any crimes to which they have been subject in the previous 12 months, irrespective of whether these offences were reported to the police. By virtue of the fact that the BCS includes both reported and unreported crimes, it is considered to be a fairer reflection – if still not a completely accurate measure – of the number of crimes in England and Wales. By comparing the BCS's figures with those of officially recorded offences, one can estimate the so-called 'dark number' of crimes; that is to say, the number of crimes that are hidden because they go unrecorded (Wilson and Ashton 1998, p. 5). The BCS does not cover all crime – for instance, corporate crime is excluded – but its latest figures for 1998 do suggest that about four times the amount of crime takes place than is indicated by the official statistics. In short, the BCS is a good indicator of the frequency of the most common crimes and how the levels of these change over time (Mirrlees-Black *et al.* 1998, p. 78).

Crime figures

While the BCS's larger figure for crime won't allay the fears of some members of the public, the BCS has tried to inject some rationality into the debate over crime and the chances of becoming a victim. Whereas police statistics may be used to compare crime rates in different police-force areas, they cannot easily demonstrate the variation in risks for different types of communities and individuals. The BCS does, however, gather data on the risks of victimization (Wasik *et al.* 1999, p. 1). The 1998 survey found that compared with property crime, the risk of becoming a victim of violence was low. Whereas, on average, 5.6% of all households in 1997 were subject to an attempted or successful burglary, only 1% of adults became the victim of a wounding (i.e. serious injury from an assault). Moreover, the highest risks of being burgled were associated with specific kinds of households with one or more of the following characteristics:

- The head of the household is young.
- The head of the household is unemployed.
- The household unit is a single family.
- The household enjoys only a low income.
- The property is rented accommodation, either privately or from the council.
- The property is left empty for 3 or more hours during the day.
- The property is a flat or is located at the end of a terrace.

Locality, too, is a factor in victimization risk. The risk of burglary is greater in an inner-city area, on a council estate, and in an area characterized by physical disorder (Mirrlees-Black *et al.* 1998, pp. 28–30).

Despite the BCS's estimate of nearly 16.5 million crimes against adults in 1997, the 1998 survey showed that there had been a fall between 1995 and 1997 in almost all categories of crimes – with burglary decreasing by 7%, violence by 17%, and thefts from vehicles by 25%. Overall, this amounted to a 14% decrease since the last BCS, which was the first occasion the survey recorded such an overall fall in crime. It also confirmed the downward trend in recent years in officially recorded crime figures (Mirrlees-Black *et al.* 1998). The decrease in violent crimes reported by the BCS can be contrasted with the 5% increase in offences involving violence against the person recorded by the police for 1997–1998. However, the police statistics also showed decreases in the number of robberies, vehicle crimes and domestic burglaries of 13%, 12% and 14% respectively. Overall, there was an 8% fall in the level of all recorded crimes – the largest of the consecutive falls in the preceding 5 years.

Despite these falls, there is still a serious crime problem in England and Wales. The official crime statistics for the period April 1997 to March 1998 indicated that 4.5 million crimes were recorded by the police (Povey and Prime 1998). Most were committed by men whose peak age for known offending was 18 (i.e. they committed the highest number of crimes in their lives when aged 18). Moreover, about 3% of offenders were estimated to have carried out approximately 25% of all offences (Home Office 1995). Furthermore, the link between drug abuse and crime has become clearer, with many crimes being committed by those needing to fuel their drug habits. Added to the high crime figures is the police's modest abilities to solve them. In 1996–1997 the average clear-up rate for all crime among the police forces in England and Wales was 24% (Audit Commission 1998b, p. 13). Furthermore, if one takes the BCS figures for the amount of crime and compares them with the official statistics for those appearing in court, it becomes clear that, 'on average, only about 2% of crimes committed actually result in a conviction' (Wasik *et al.* 1999, p. 7).

CRIME, FEAR OF CRIME AND MORAL PANICS

There has never been a Golden Age in which crime rates were so low that citizens had little or no fear of crime and in which friendly bobbies patrolled their patch keeping order and providing help in a paternalistic fashion. Yet, many people look back nostalgically to an age when property crime and violence were much lower. I remember that when living in South Wales in the 1950s, it was common to leave one's front-door key under the door mat, so slight was the expectation that one might be burgled. The perception that one's community was a relatively safe place persisted in the minds of many people during the

1950s, despite the fact that crime had already begun to grow rapidly. This is not the place to enquire in detail as to why so much more crime occurs today than in the 1950s, but certainly society has undergone a startling transformation in the intervening decades – and especially between 1979 and 1992, when recorded offences rose from 2.4 million to 5.4 million (James and Raine 1998, p. 6). Moreover, 'current levels of recorded crime are nearly 10 times greater than the level of recorded crime in the 1950s' (Wasik *et al.* 1999, p. 4). The 1992 figure was the highest ever figure for officially recorded crime and each year since there have been small decreases in the number of officially recorded crimes. During this period, 1992 to 1998, the decreases in overall crime and the specific decline in property crimes have been accompanied by increases in the level of officially recorded violent crime.

The social changes of the 1960s and 1970s ushered in a new concern for crime and for social order. Whereas previously major legislation on crime had been relatively rare, the 1980s and 1990s have seen a dramatic increase in laws related to crime, policing and criminal justice policies. Not only have governments focused more firmly on criminal justice issues, but the public and the press have also become more vocal in their demands to stem what is increasingly being perceived as a tidal wave of crime sweeping the nation. For much of the last two decades England and Wales have been engaged in a 'war on crime' and, as it has become clear that the war is not being won, so the criticisms of the criminal justice system have grown. Indeed, at times, crime has become so emotive an issue, that it has been elevated to the status of a moral panic, and consequently many people wildly overestimate their chances of becoming a victim. This further increases the fear of crime and fuels the moral panic even more, especially as the media exaggerate the chances of falling victim to violent or sexual crime (Wasik *et al.* 1999, p. 1). In the war on crime all the criminal justice agencies were required to become more effective, and new technology (such as CCTV in city centres, car parks and shopping arcades) was enthusiastically embraced. Ironically, even as technology was introduced, many criminal justice organizations – especially the police, the courts and the prisons – found themselves almost overwhelmed by the number of people and cases they had to process (James and Raine 1998, p. 6).

Risk assessment and victimization

Although the 1998 BCS noted a drop in the levels of concern among the public concerning crime (especially in relation to burglary and car crime), the levels are still high. About a fifth of the BCS's respondents reported that they were very worried about a range of crimes. Of women in the sample, 31% said that they were very worried about the possibility of rape, and inner-city dwellers had more concern about all types of crime than those living elsewhere; 11% of people reported that they felt very unsafe out alone after dark and another 21% said they felt fairly unsafe. These figures cannot be divorced from people's knowledge and perception of crime. If the public sees crime as more prevalent than it is, this will contribute to the sense of unease. In fact, this is just what the 1998 BCS found – the public in general tend to over-estimate the crime problem. Although the levels of police-recorded crime and the levels reported in the BCS both fell between 1995 and 1997, only 9% of people were aware of it. Moreover, whereas the BCS showed that around 20% of crime was violent, 58% of respondents believed that violent crime amounted to at least half the total (Mirrlees-Black and Allen 1998). On a related matter, official police-recorded figures for 1997–1998 showed that violent crime – defined as violence against the person, sexual offences and robbery – amounted to 8% of all offences recorded by the police (Povey and Prime 1998).

Fear of crime is not always irrational. Many people live in areas where they have good reason to be fearful. The more crime there is in one's neighbourhood, the more one will have good reason to be fearful of crime. However, those who believe themselves to be at greatest risk are mistaken. Older people as a group, for example, have no reason to be so fearful of crime since they are at relatively low risk of becoming its victim. It is young, socially active men who run the greatest risk, because of their behaviour and lifestyle. They are out drinking a great deal, leaving their homes unoccupied, and so are likely to become victims of violence and of burglary. The chances of becoming a victim are not, therefore, equally distributed. The risk of becoming a victim of burglary is greater in an inner-city area than in the countryside. Members of ethnic minority groups are more likely to become victims of crime in general than white people. Women and children are much more at risk of violence in the home than elderly people.

While violent crime has generally been increasing, it is still only a small proportion of all recorded crime; but, once again, the chances of becoming a victim are not equally distributed. Approximately two-thirds of the victims of violent crime between 1990 and 1994 were male, the majority being aged between 16 and 39. The elderly enjoy a relatively low risk of becoming a victim of any form of violence. However, the position of women and ethnic minorities is different. Almost 50% of violent offences against women took place in their own homes or in the suspects' homes, which reflects the 'greater "domestic" nature of violence against women' (Watson 1996, p. 1). Members of ethnic minorities are at greater risk of becoming victims on two counts. First, they tend, on average, to be younger, to be poorer, and to live in higher-risk urban areas – all of which increase the chances of becoming a victim. Second, they are additionally subject to racially motivated crimes, which amount to about 15% of crimes committed against them. Accordingly, ethnic minorities tend to have a greater fear of crime than white people (Percy 1998).

Moral panic versus reality

At the heart of people's fears about crime, and upon which many media stories dwell, is the fear of being attacked by a stranger in completely random circumstances – an attack against which, of course, it would be virtually impossible to protect oneself. Unfortunately, it is only recently that we have started to apply a more rational analysis to the crime problem in general and random attacks in particular. One example of this was the Home Office minister, Lord Williams of Mostyn, who admitted in October 1998 that previous government policy on violent crime had been designed in ignorance of the true extent and nature of this type of offence (*The Independent*, 20 October 1998, p. 5). In the same month a major study of violent crime was launched by the Economic and Social Research Council (ESRC). Its preliminary findings were completely at odds with the notion, often implied by the media and politicians, that the public were at serious risk of random attacks by complete strangers. On the contrary, violence by a stranger is the rarest form of violence, and people are much more likely to be assaulted and even murdered by relatives, spouses and those with whom they work. Moreover, most violence occurs according to well-known patterns – men attacking men in public places and women and children being abused at home. The ESRC study will doubtless want to look in more detail at the figures for violent crime in order to ascertain whether the official increase in such figures is due to people's greater readiness to report crimes of violence to the police, to changes in the manner in which the police record such offences, or to a real increase in violence (*The Guardian*, 20 October 1998, p. 8).

The moral panic about crime, especially violent crime, has been strengthened throughout the 1980s and 1990s by associated public anxieties over urban disorder, children seemingly out of control, burgeoning drug use, hooliganism, vandalism and terrorism (James and Raine 1998, p. 6). The matter has not been helped by the increase in violent offences among teenage females who now commit about one in four juvenile crimes, as opposed to one in eleven in 1957. In the period 1988 to 1998, the number of arrests of girls for violent crimes has doubled and teenage-female crime is now increasing at a faster rate than that of boys. Reasons for this change may be the greater time that girls now spend outside the home, the decrease in direct parental supervision and the increased tendency of girls to hang around the streets with groups of other girls or with boys. In short, in some respects, the adolescent behaviour of girls is becoming more similar to that of boys (*The Daily Telegraph*, 16 October 1998, pp. 1–2). No wonder, therefore, that crime and the fear of crime are serious social problems in England and Wales today. What, then, is the response of the state to the problem of crime?

THE RESPONSE OF THE CRIMINAL JUSTICE AGENCIES

Even if the public were not fearful about crime, the state would still have to respond to it. In the first place, crime runs counter to our sense of moral values and all societies adopt various ways of sanctioning inappropriate activities. Second, burgeoning criminal activity, if left unchecked, might pose a threat to the continuation of civilized, democratic society. However, this does not mean that we must inevitably adopt draconian measures to combat crime, for under our system of justice people are innocent until proven guilty and therefore are entitled to a number of rights. On the contrary, a civilized and democratic country will adopt reason-able measures that maintain a balance between the need to fight crime, to protect citizens and to punish criminals on the one hand, and the necessity to uphold civil liberties and to provide a humane system of criminal justice on the other. Nor need our criminal justice system be rigidly applied. Justice demands that, in certain circumstances, the full weight of the law be tempered. Thus, juvenile delinquents are treated differently, but not unfairly, because of their age and because society has long recognized that special care is required when the criminal justice system is handling young people. Equally, society and our system of justice acknowledge that not all crimes are the same, nor deserving of the same punishments. The woman who defends herself against a violent attack by her partner and in so doing inflicts serious harm upon her attacker is rightly treated differently from someone who callously and premeditatedly causes harm to another.

The agencies of the criminal justice system are the major response of the state to crime. Their main tasks are:

- to detect and prosecute those suspected of criminal acts
- to provide and administer justice in accordance with the due process of law
- to protect the public from crime and criminals
- to provide a range of penalties and sentences for those convicted of crime
- to attempt to rehabilitate criminals.

The detection of crime and its investigation has long been one of the primary responsibilities of the police. This in itself has an important element of public protection, which is again evident when the police are involved in suppressing public disorder, such as rioting and looting. The prosecution of defendants is carried out by the Crown Prosecution Service (CPS) which, together with the Youth Court and the adult courts, is responsible for the provision and administration of justice in England and Wales. Defence lawyers, often provided through the Legal Aid scheme at public expense, are another vital aspect in the provision of justice. The courts and the CPS also provide an element of public protection when dangerous or persistent offenders are sentenced to imprisonment. The prison and probation services provide many of the penalties available to the courts, but it is the courts themselves that collect any fines which sentencers have awarded. (The government proposed in November 1998 that in future the collection of fines and the power to make arrests for unpaid fines might be delegated to the private sector, much to the concern of legal and civil rights agencies.) Helping people to turn away from a criminal career has historically been the responsibility of the prisons and the probation service, although nowadays the rehabilitative efforts within prison have been much reduced in favour of its growing focus on public protection through the incapacitation (i.e. removal from society) of offenders. Indeed, probation officers now pursue more of a public-protection role through their recent focus on risk assessment and the administration of community penalties. Finally, since the passing of the Crime and Disorder Act 1998, with its emphasis on local partnerships to fight crime, local councils are becoming involved with other agencies to implement policies to make towns and cities safer places in which to live (James and Raine 1998, pp. 9–10).

CONCLUSION

Crime, alongside poverty, poor housing, ill-health and unemployment is one of this country's biggest social problems. As with all social problems, governments introduce a variety of policies and support a number of different agencies to try to alleviate the problem. In the case of crime, special care must be taken both with the policies and the agencies to ensure that they do not become draconian. It is a difficult and constantly changing task to strike the right balance between what are often conflicting demands. On the one hand, elements of public and political opinion (and perhaps victims more than anyone else) may demand stiffer penalties, while the police may call for greater powers and fewer safeguards for suspects. On the other hand, suspects and defendants and even prisoners still have certain rights and these cannot be ignored – otherwise we slip into authoritarianism. The task is not made easier by the general level of ignorance among public, media and politicians concerning the extent of crime and the groups most at risk of victimization. Exercises such as the BCS and the officially recorded statistics adopt a more rational and wholly unsensational approach to the crime problem and have the potential to make an educational impact on all concerned. Instead of a moral panic about crime, we can then move towards an informed debate.

As can be seen, some of the tasks of the criminal justice system are shared by various agencies. (For an overview of the work and aims of the main agencies in the criminal justice system, see Chapter 4.) However, the work of the criminal justice system begins with the police; and it is to a detailed consideration of that organization that we turn next.

KEY POINTS

- Much crime is associated with poverty and changes within the economy.
- In 1998 both official police-recorded crime and the levels of crime reported as part of the BCS fell.
- Fear of crime is still significant, and most people are either ignorant of the extent of crime or overestimate their own chances of becoming a victim.
- Not everyone is at equal risk of becoming a victim. The elderly are a low-risk group while young males are high risk. Inner-city dwellers are at more risk that those who live in the countryside.
- Violent crime is still only a small proportion of all crime, but it receives disproportionate media attention.

GUIDE TO FURTHER READING

In Chapter 1 of Wasik, M., Gibbons, T. and Redmayne, M. (1999) *Criminal Justice. Text and Materials,* London: Longman, there is coverage of crime statistics and the nature of the crime problem, and on pp. 167–174 measures of crime, such as the BCS, and the extent of crime are dealt with.

The problem of crime and the role of criminal justice agencies are dealt with in Chapter 1 of James, A. and Raine, J. (1998) *The New Politics of Criminal Justice,* London: Longman.

Images of crime, crime as a social problem, victimization, the impact of crime, and measures of crime are dealt with in Chapters 2 and 3 of Davies, M., Croall, H. and Tyrer, J. (1998) *Criminal Justice. An Introduction to the Criminal Justice System in England and Wales.* 2nd edition, London: Longman.

Free from the Home Office is Mirrlees-Black, C., Budd, T., Partridge, S. and Mayhew, P. (1998) *The 1998 British Crime Survey. England and Wales,* Home Office Statistical Bulletin, London. Despite its statistical bulletin label, this is an easy-to-read account of the extent of crime, trends in crime, and the nature of victimization.

Chapter 1 of Muncie, J. and McLaughlin, E. (eds) (1996) *The Problem of Crime,* Beverley Hills, CA: Sage, explains what crime is, how it is reported and how it is measured.

The police service: putting care first

2

Outline
- Over many years the police have been reorganized and reduced to their present number of 43 constabularies.
- The police deploy many specialist units and take advantage of many sophisticated technological aids.
- Police activities often have a dual 'care' and 'control' purpose.
- Examples of the caring approach are community policing and neighbourhood watch. The handling of the mentally ill and the recruitment of women and ethnic minorities to the police have created the potential for a caring approach but there are currently several difficulties in achieving this.
- The police 'canteen culture' is not generally sympathetic to a more caring approach.

THE HISTORY AND DEVELOPMENT OF THE POLICE

The modern police service owes its origins to Sir Robert Peel and his creation of the Metropolitan Police in London in 1829. After this date, other towns followed suit and by 1856 all counties in England and Wales were required by law to set up a police force (Stead 1985). During the nineteenth century, over 200 police forces came into existence and in 1939 (despite a few amalgamations) there were still 183 constabularies. These constabularies employed 60,000 officers in total, but only 200 were women (who had only been allowed to join the service during the First World War). Since then, as a result of legislation and a number of mergers, the number of police forces has been drastically reduced. On 31 March 1998, the police constabularies of England and Wales could be described in general terms as follows.

- The number of constabularies amounted to 43.
- The total number of officers employed by the 43 constabularies was 124,798.

- 16% of officers were women.
- 2% of officers came from ethnic minorities.
- An additional 2,000 officers were seconded to regional crime squads and other inter-force agencies (Prime *et al.* 1998).
- In 1997–1998 the police service cost over £7 billion a year (Audit Commission 1998b).

The objectives of the fledgling Metropolitan Police were the prevention of crime, the preservation of the peace, and the detection of offenders. It was not long before these last two objectives became paramount, with crime prevention taking something of a back seat (Newburn 1995; Stead 1985). Indeed, the order maintenance capabilities of the police were greatly enhanced by the fact that they were originally set up along quasi-military lines with a hierarchy of ranks, a distinctive uniform, centralized 'top-down' control, and strict regulations governing the behaviour of officers.

Initially, the introduction of the 'new' police (called 'bobbies' after Sir Robert Peel) encountered a great deal of public hostility (Newburn 1995, p. 43), but, on the whole, the police in England and Wales have operated with quite strong public approval – the basis of the so-called 'British police advantage'. The 1996 British Crime Survey found that 81% of the public thought that their local police did a very or fairly good job (Mirrlees-Black and Budd 1997). Of course, there have been periods when the police and the public have been engaged in outright animosity. However, the post-war period and the 1950s were the high point of policing by consent – during which time the police were able to adopt a more consciously peacekeeping role than is the case today. This period is symbolized by that fictional television character, Dixon of Dock Green, who patrolled his beat with paternal concern for those who lived there (Reiner 1985; Newburn 1995). This was a time when there was much less crime, and both society and the police were far less mobile. Police and public could get to know one another as officers patrolled their regular beats on foot; frequently they shared similar values. The public accorded greater respect to the police constable than is the case today, and the officer took a good deal of occupational satisfaction in carrying out the peacekeeping role (Banton 1973). (How this predominantly peacekeeping role with its elements of care and service became once again strongly rooted in law enforcement and order maintenance is explained in Chapter 3.)

With the exception of the Metropolitan Police and the City of London Police, constabularies have much in common. They have the same rank structure; they are accountable to local police authorities composed of elected councillors, JPs and other local people; and they are organized in much the same way. Each police force (including both of those in London) is divided into divisions, sub-divisions or sectors (or whatever local term is used to describe this geographical locality), which are used as administrative, operational and specific beat or patrol bases. Moreover, all constabularies are further organized according to specialism. While patrol officers (usually of constable rank) may be the largest specialism, there are also many others including CID, traffic division, dog patrols, drug-squad officers, control-room officers, custody officers, personnel involved in training, and so on. In addition, the police employ over 56,000 civilians to carry out non-operational duties, and there are also over 18,000 special constables (part-time volunteers) who go on patrol and undertake other duties to supplement the work of paid, full-time police officers (Prime *et al.* 1998). However, in recent years, despite greater funding and a political desire to increase the number of police officers, their ranks have diminished. In the year ending March 1999, the number of officers fell to 123,922.

Whereas the original bobby on patrol had only a rattle or a whistle with which to summon help and only a wooden truncheon with which to defend himself, the modern police officer has a myriad of technology on which to call. Special clothing and equipment are available to provide protection during episodes of public disorder; the wooden truncheon has been replaced by the high-tech extendible baton, and officers also carry CS gas sprays; personal radios are used not only to summon help instantly but also to request information; powerful computers check a range of data and provide answers to questions from officers on patrol; and new kinds of technology such as DNA testing are regularly being used by the police. Modern officers and their equipment are very different from those who walked London's streets back in the nineteenth century. Yet both sets of officers would still recognize the essentially similar organizational and rank structures, as well as the major operational objectives of the police. However, despite these similarities across time and between current police forces, it would be a mistake to view the police as a monolithic organization. As we shall see later in this chapter and in Chapter 3, in cultural terms there is not a single police organization, but several. It is the nature of the rank structure itself and the sometimes unsympathetic feeling between officers in different specialisms that makes this so.

For much of the period of the Conservative Government between 1979 and 1997 the police enjoyed a generous level of state financing in terms of improved salary levels, increases in staff numbers, and greater technological resources. However, even the Conservative Government eventually became sceptical of the typical police rallying cry of 'give us more personnel and resources and we will reduce crime' (Morgan and Newburn 1997, pp. 46-50). The Labour Government that came to power in May 1997 has taken this a stage further. It proposed that the police should face a strict efficiency drive as part of the government's plans to introduce a new crime-prevention strategy, much of which is contained in the Crime and Disorder Act 1998. Although the government pledged extra funding to the police over the period 1998–2001, this will be accompanied by improved efficiency targets of 2% per annum with the extra savings being re-directed into front-line policing priorities.

This will mean many changes in the way the police work. There will be a new focus on 'what works' in terms of reducing or preventing crime. Empirical evidence suggests that simply putting more bobbies on the beat does little to reduce crime. Similarly ineffective are neighbourhood watch and random patrolling. Accordingly, the police are to concentrate more firmly on what does work, such as targeting repeat offenders using intelligence-led policing, directed patrolling at crime hot spots, targeting repeat victims, and problem-oriented policing. However, while a policy such as zero tolerance policing may cut crime in a small area in the short term, its long-term effects are not yet clear. The Crime and Disorder Act 1998 will require the police not only to adopt a variety of new measures, but also to tailor their responses to the needs of particular areas after public consultation concerning policing priorities.

CARE AND CONTROL

The police force is a complex organization. Constabularies share many things in common, but each constabulary will also have organizational fault-lines running, in large measure, along the axes of rank and specialism. However, in general, the work the police perform has either a caring or a controlling function (Stephens and Becker 1994). With complex phenomena the tendency is to reduce them to stereotypes, but the division between these two functions is not as straightforward as it might seem. A village bobby talking to villagers is likely to be seen as an example of the caring approach, and officers in military-style uniform rushing headlong into a crowd and wielding their batons to be viewed as the ultimate instance of control. These actions may often be straightforward examples of each approach, but not always. The village bobby may be talking to a friend about the whereabouts of someone he wishes to arrest and take away for questioning – a clear control issue. The police riot squad may be protecting the rights – indeed the safety – of a minority group who have been set upon by those hostile to them – an example of caring for others even though force has been used. In short, care and control are not always separate matters, but frequently overlap so that a matrix of care and control is formed out of the totality of police activities (Stephens and Becker 1994). There are many duties carried out by the police that contain elements of both approaches, but one can usually identify whether the activity is predominantly related to the caring approach or to the controlling. In this chapter, the detailed examples of police activities relate primarily to the caring approach, while Chapter 3 sets out examples of the controlling approach.

Modern policing emphasizes the controlling approach, especially among the lower ranks that comprise the strongest elements of the 'canteen culture'. This term refers to the unofficial culture of the lower ranks that prizes commonsense, physical presence, and 'getting the bloody job done' above what they often perceive as the fanciful notions of policy-planning and implementation, intellectual rigour, and ethical behaviour. The canteen culture is immensely strong and shared (to lesser or greater degrees) by most officers among the lower ranks. The terms used to summarize types of control are law enforcement, crime control and order maintenance. Maintaining order is closely associated with the police presence at sporting events, demonstrations and marches. Restoring public order is something that the police are not frequently called upon to perform – at least not usually on any large scale over a significant period of time. Law enforcement is another example of control, even though it, too, contains elements of the caring approach. For example, preventing someone from becoming a repeat burglary-victim through some form of police action or intervention contains clear elements of both.

Despite these major controlling functions, much of what the police do is routine and not crime-related. Non-crime-related activities are called the 'service function' of the police and have affinities with the caring approach (Punch 1979). Included here would be examples of the police giving advice to people concerning all kinds of ordinary difficulties, and even talking to those people who stop for a social chat with officers (Mirrlees-Black and Budd 1997). The mundane and, in many officers' eyes, boring aspects of the service function are the bedrock of policing, despite television dramas that depict unusual occurrences, acts of violence and general mayhem as if they were commonplace.

Two major operational examples of police activities that are predominantly oriented towards a caring approach are community policing (and its related 'sub-species' of neighbourhood watch), and the partnership approach with other agencies, especially local authorities, to prevent crime. However, the handling of the mentally ill and the recruitment of women and ethnic minorities to the force are areas where a more caring approach has frequently been absent.

POLICE WORK AND THE CARING APPROACH: SUCCESSES AND FAILURES

Community policing and neighbourhood watch

Community policing has been described as a 'softly, softly' and more proactive approach to crime, and as a necessary alternative to the sometimes abrasive tactics deployed as part of the law-enforcement or reactive approach (Alderson 1979). This latter approach reacts to crime incidents, perhaps by deploying CID personnel if the crime is sufficiently serious, or by deploying squads of uniformed officers as part of a 'stop and search' tactic. Community policing is more proactive and usually has a specific geographical focus (Gilling 1996, pp. 105–6). In broad terms, it may be summarized as follows.

- Community policing seeks to strengthen public confidence and trust in the police.
- It tries to improve communication between the police and the public, and, hence, to increase public co-operation – especially in relation to gaining crime-related information.
- It has a distinct crime prevention focus, and is designed to be a form of more publicly acceptable policing.

These characteristics are necessary because frequently 'the police emphasise the detection of crime rather than its prevention. In too many forces crime prevention is a relatively low-status, poorly resourced activity' (Audit Commission 1993, p. 14). Community policing is often seen as promoting 'generalist patrol-based skills', as opposed to the specialist duties of other kinds of officers (Fielding 1995, p. 200).

At the heart of community policing is the idea of the police and public (and other agencies, if necessary) working in partnership. However, forms of community policing vary enormously, and range from a single officer walking a regular beat, to multi-agency co-ordination to tackle social deprivation and associated deviancy in a particular area. Included in that range is neighbourhood watch.

Like community policing schemes in general, neighbourhood watch has both a crime prevention purpose and one intended to reduce fear of crime. For instance, members of neighbourhood-watch schemes are supposed to benefit not only from neighbours being the extra ears and eyes of the police and reporting suspicious events to them, but are also supposed to feel safer from the threat of burglary and other crimes precisely because neighbours are helping to protect one another. Ideally, neighbourhood watch schemes should foster a sense among their members that community watchfulness, combined with police support, can help to reduce crime and improve crime prevention. Indeed, many thousands of such schemes have been set up over the years. However, various empirical studies suggest that they are not successful. McConville and Shepherd (1992, p. 115) refer to neighbourhood watch as suffering from 'low take-up rates, weak community penetration and limping, dormant or stillborn schemes'. Turner and Alexandrou (1997) found that although neighbourhood watch schemes were seen by their civilian co-ordinators as a way of helping the police, these co-ordinators were dissatisfied with the levels of communication, support and feedback from the police – which they took to be indicative of the police's generally poor attitude to such schemes. The police themselves generally supported the concept of neighbourhood watch, but had strong doubts about whether these schemes delivered any effective benefit. Moreover, even officers who welcomed neighbourhood watch were unsure how to maintain effective lines of communication between themselves and scheme members. Finally, Jordan (1998, p. 68) in a review of several pieces of research on neighbourhood watch concluded that the schemes fared best in areas of relative affluence with low crime-rates and least well in areas with high crime-rates. In short, they had little effect in preventing crime nationally.

As Fielding (1995) points out, the failure of one form of community policing – in this case, neighbourhood watch – does not mean that community policing as a whole is without merit. On the contrary, it means that in order to evaluate the effectiveness of community policing we need to look in detail at each example of the genre. Jordan (1998) has highlighted a number of community-oriented strategies that may have value. Whereas neighbourhood watch fails to engage the majority of people living in high-crime areas, it may be that community participation in setting priorities for police action and responses will be able to achieve that goal. Here, the role of community constable would become as important as that of specialist officers because the former would attempt to ensure the direct participation of the public in consultative meetings with local CID and other specialist squads, as well as being in a position to pass on information about crime and the public's preferences for police action. Another strategy that may be worth pursuing with a community policing aspect is that of problem-oriented policing (POP).

POP is about solving the underlying problems of an area and not simply reacting to crime calls. For such a strategy to work, officers must have a detailed knowledge of those underlying problems; have regular contacts with the community; have information to help them understand the community's problems and the way in which those problems may manifest themselves as clusters of criminal activities; and be supported by senior officers (Jordan 1998, p. 73). Moreover, any successful implemen-tation of POP would have to overcome any cultural resistance on the part of officers to this new way of working (Leigh *et al.* 1998). Although POP is little tried in this country and is not without its difficulties, the overall approach is one that would fit comfortably within a community policing approach and (with the right support and training) might serve to re-energize police attitudes towards this form of policing. However, it must be acknowledged that current evidence suggests that most forms of community policing and neighbourhood watch, while they may help to reduce fear of crime, do little to reduce crime itself, or to improve crime prevention.

The partnership approach

In some respects, this approach is a continuation of community policing, since it also adopts a proactive position in respect of crime and has the clear objective of improving crime prevention. As the name implies, the police forge a partnership in the fight against crime. Even before 1998 many police forces emphasized that they could not fight crime alone and that they needed the help of the public. Following the Crime and Disorder Act 1998, the partnership has been extended to include not just the public but also other organizations and agencies – the most important of which are local authorities. The police, local authorities and other agencies, such as the probation and local health services, are required to carry out the following statutory duties (Hough and Tilley 1998):

- conduct and publish a local audit of crime and disorder
- consult with the public and other organizations in relation to the audit's findings
- set district-based targets for a reduction in crime and incidences of disorder
- monitor the progress made towards achieving those targets
- repeat this process every 3 years.

Although the police and local authorities are now statutorily required to form a crime prevention partnership, local people are also supposed to play their part. The government feels that the Crime and Disorder Act 1998 will help to empower people in the fight against crime. For instance, neighbourhood watch is intended to play a key role (Turner and Alexandrou 1997). Members of neighbourhood watch groups might make ready targets for public consultation concerning the findings of the crime and disorder audit and be in a position to voice their concerns about local patterns of crime and how the police and other agencies should respond. It is even envisaged that these same groups might develop a greater emphasis on self-help activities, such as assisting with youth diversion schemes, reducing fear of crime and building up community spirit. However, such a vision of the future role of neighbourhood watch is probably over-ambitious and beyond the capacity and commitment of most groups. Given the general failure of neighbourhood watch, its key role will have to be critically rethought, and new forms of support and organization will have to follow if neighbourhood watch is to play an effective role in the partnership.

Although strategies to reduce crime and disorder must be driven by those things that matter to local people, it is difficult to see how the public can be actively involved beyond being consulted. It will be panels of experts and professionals who will draw up strategies and, for the most part, implement them. The police fear that they will be automatically cast as the lead agency in local partnerships designed to combat crime. They would prefer that once the local causes of crime and disorder have been uncovered they be addressed by the most appropriate agencies; for instance, by the utility company to improve local lighting conditions in a particular area if this is shown to be a causal factor in incidences of crime and disorder. Clearly, the consequences of the Crime and Disorder Act 1998 will be to create a variety of different, locally-based partnerships but it remains to be seen whether the Act will also usher in a new kind of activist citizenry, full of volunteering zeal to take practical measures to counter crime. When all is said and done, it is still large agencies such as the police and local authorities that have the resources to tackle crime and that are, therefore, likely to be the major partners in any joint initiative. However, the public's consultative role could mean that those resources will become better targeted and lead to more effective outcomes.

Police handling of the mentally ill

The police are a 24-hour emergency service, dealing with all manner of incidents. In recent years, largely as a result of the inability of the community care system properly to support the needs of mentally ill people living in the community, the police have had to deal with an increasing number of cases involving mental health crises. The manner in which the police respond to such incidents is an example of the combination of care and control inherent in this line of work. Many individuals with continuing mental health problems who fail to receive adequate help from community-based treatment facilities may 'destabilize' and manifest behaviour that brings them to the attention of the police. If a police officer believes an individual is suffering from a mental illness, the officer may remove that person to a place of safety (such as a mental hospital or a police station) using the powers granted by Section 136 of the Mental Health Act 1983. The purpose of this procedure is to allow for the psychiatric evaluation of the individual detained under Section 136.

On the whole, the police do not much like this kind of work, because 'handling mentals' is not often considered proper police work (Murphy 1986; Teplin 1984). Moreover, several critics have pointed to the over-concentration of black people detained under Section 136 as evidence of possible racial discrimination by the police (Bean *et al.* 1991). On the other hand, police officers are quite competent at identifying someone who is mentally ill and accordingly use Section 136 wherever possible, as opposed to arresting the individual on a criminal charge and thus risking that the individual might end up being processed by the criminal justice system when immediate psychiatric help is what is required (Stephens and Becker 1994).

The handling of the mentally ill, therefore, contains clear elements of both care and control; indeed, some elements of control may have degenerated to the extent that they are examples of racial bias. However, the fact that many individuals failed by the community care system nevertheless come to receive medical help is indicative of the caring aspect of Section 136. What is needed, however, to ensure that the caring aspect is accentuated still further is the provision of crisis intervention services, such as operate in parts of the USA (Stephens 1994a and 1994b). Crisis intervention services take advantage of the police's case-finding role in which many cases involving the mentally ill are referred to them by the public. When the police are called to such a case and the officers determine that the individual is suffering a mental disturbance, they can call for immediate assistance from the crisis intervention service. Indeed, in many cases the police can hand over the individual to the mental health staff of the crisis service for evaluation and subsequent treatment, which allows the officers to return more swiftly to their crime-fighting duties. This arrangement suits both the cultural expectations of the police (who frequently prefer to engage in their law enforcement role) and the needs of the individual to receive medical help, and enables both the police and the crisis service to fulfil a caring role. In the absence of such crisis services in this country, the caring role of the police in helping the mentally ill will remain underdeveloped and open to potential abuse.

The recruitment of women and ethnic minority police officers

The police have not been pioneers in the recruitment of women and ethnic minorities. Indeed, even today, when many improvements in the field of equal opportunities, racial awareness and discrimination have been achieved, the police are still regularly criticized for both sexist and racist attitudes. The main reason for recruiting more women and people from ethnic minorities is to make the police more representative and understanding of the people they serve.

On the whole, women have fared somewhat better than ethnic minority officers. The proportion of women in the force has increased from around 12% 10 years ago to 16% today, and currently two chief constables are female. Between April 1997 and March 1998 over 25% of new officers recruited to the police were female (Prime *et al.* 1998, p. 1). Women officers also now carry out more or less the same duties as their male colleagues. However, the majority of women are still concentrated in the lower ranks. As at 31 March 1998, only 6% of assistant chief constables were female, compared with 18% of constables. In fact, 91% of all serving female officers held the rank of constable, as opposed to 75% of male officers. The proportions of female officers among the middle ranks of police management – inspector, chief inspector and superintendent – were 5%, 6% and 4% respectively. Nearly 95% of officers holding the rank of inspector or above were male (Prime *et al.* 1998, p. 2). In addition, there are regular and sometimes unseemly public revelations of sexist attitudes among some male officers, accompanied by sex discrimination cases being taken to tribunals by female officers alleging that their careers have been damaged in one way or another.

Although individual female officers are fighting to gain improvements in the treatment of all women in the police, and the police organization itself is also trying to improve its equal opportunities record, much more still needs to be done, as the wastage figures for female officers clearly indicate. Whereas in the year up to 31 March 1998 of all male officers leaving the police 74% retired, 12% resigned and 14% left for other reasons, in the case of female officers these proportions were 45% retired, 33% resigned and 22% left for other reasons (Prime *et al.* 1998, p. 4). The high percentage of women resigning from the organization suggests a strong level of dissatisfaction with or problems in the job.

Improvements in the lot of ethnic minority officers is slower, although the publicity surrounding racial issues is equally pronounced and regularly causes additional embarrassment to the police hierarchy. In 1984 less than 1% of the police were drawn from ethnic minorities. As a result of a number of recruiting campaigns, by 1994 this had increased to 1.5% and as at 31 March

1998 it stood at 2% (Home Office 1998e). To reflect the proportion of ethnic minorities in the UK population as a whole it should be close to 6% – and much higher than that in cities such as London, Leicester, Bradford, and so on. Of the 2,483 ethnic minority officers in the police forces of England and Wales in March 1998, 88% were constables (Prime *et al.* 1998, pp. 1 and 5). Many commentators and members of ethnic minorities themselves have suggested that the low recruitment figures reflect the general unwillingness of black and Asian people to join an organization that they perceive as racist. In 1999 the government announced that all police forces would have to meet targets, roughly in line with the proportions of ethnic minorities within their constabulary boundaries, for recruiting significantly higher numbers of ethnic minority officers. Some police forces will be faced with very challenging targets to meet in the next few years and it will be instructive to note how they go about their task, what support the government provides, and how the government will react if these targets are not fulfilled.

In addition, there is the whole business of the alleged racism of white officers not only towards their non-white colleagues, but also towards black and Asian members of the public. Following the controversy surrounding the inquiry into the murder of the young black man Stephen Lawrence, and the manner in which the Metropolitan Police handled their investigation, there was an unprecedented number of twelve chief constables who subsequently admitted to various forms of racism within their own constabularies; two of them also acknowledged the existence of institutional racism (*The Independent*, 16 October 1998, p. 1). Such an incidence of racism has, of course, nothing to do with a caring approach, but falls firmly into the controlling area which we will turn to in the next chapter.

CONCLUSION

There are two major difficulties that would have to be overcome if a more effective and predominantly caring approach were to be implemented. First, the police are heavily committed to a law enforcement and order maintenance style of policing and they do not always accept nor fully understand how other tactics, more in keeping with a caring approach, could achieve the goals of controlling crime and maintaining the peace. Their overly optimistic attachment to technological advances also underpins this perspective. Second, there is an exceptionally strong 'macho' element within the police, especially among the lower ranks which are dominated by male constables. Added to this is the presence of a significant racist element. The canteen culture in the police frequently stands opposed to that emanating from various specialist squads and from senior management in particular. Rules may be bent or circumvented to suit the needs, values and norms of the canteen culture and this can make it very difficult for senior officers to bring about change. Worse still is the fact that the canteen culture may place expectations on officers not to co-operate with inquiries concerning police corruption. These matters are considered in more detail in Chapter 3 where the nature of the controlling approach in police work is examined.

KEY POINTS

- Although hierarchical and bureaucratic, the police force is not monolithic but has many specialisms and is a complex organization.
- Its primary roles are law enforcement and order maintenance, with a more recent focus on crime prevention.
- Police activities divide into those with a predominantly caring or controlling element, which together form a matrix of care and control.
- Examples of the caring approach are community policing, neighbourhood watch, and the partnership approach.
- Activities where a caring approach is under-developed or has failed include the handling of the mentally ill, and the recruitment of women and ethnic minority officers.
- The canteen culture is the biggest obstacle facing the implementation of a more caring approach.
- Although they may help to reduce fear of crime, most current forms of community policing and neighbourhood watch do little to reduce crime or improve prevention.

GUIDE TO FURTHER READING

An explanation of the care and control argument, as well as examples of 'caring' police activities, is provided in Stephens, M. and Becker, S. (1994) *Police Force, Police Service. Care and Control in Britain.* London: Macmillan.

For a detailed and closely argued account of the benefits and difficulties associated with community policing, see Fielding, N. (1995) *Community Policing*, Oxford: Clarendon Press.

There is an excellent account of racial issues within the police written by someone who has an intimate knowledge of the field in Holdaway, S. (1996) *The Racialisation of British Policing*, London: Macmillan. This is also very useful for Chapter 3.

For a review and assessment of the latest evidence concerning what works in reducing offending, see Home Office (1998a) *Reducing Offending. An Assessment of Research Evidence on Ways of Dealing with Offending Behaviour*, Home Office Research Study 187, London. Chapter 6 deals with police strategies to reduce crime.

A detailed account of the development of the police can be found in Emsley, C. (1996) *The English Police: A Political and Social History*, 2nd edition, Longman.

The police force: being in control

3

Outline
- The culture of control is still very strong in the police.
- Examples of the controlling approach are stop and search, paramilitary activities, intelligence-led operations, and zero tolerance.
- The existence of police racism and overreliance on stereotyping leads to harassment of and discrimination against ethnic minorities.
- The employment of more female and ethnic-minority officers could help to overcome some of the above problems.

THE CONTROLLING APPROACH

The police are the ultimate civil authority for maintaining and, especially, restoring public order; beyond them is the army. The inception of the police was linked to a period of both rapid industrialization and social change in which the growing ranks of the urban poor, the so-called 'dangerous classes', posed a threat to the status quo. The police were set up to handle that threat, to maintain order, and to clamp down on increasing lawlessness especially in the poorer areas. From its earliest days, therefore, the police force has placed great emphasis on its order maintenance and law enforcement (crime control) duties. Ironically, despite this initial emphasis, relatively little police time and resources are now expended on these activities. In 1971, for example, as much as 80% of public calls to the police were non-crime-related. The Audit Commission reported in 1993 that:

> about 60 per cent of calls to a police station were not related to crime but to personal difficulties and problems, noise disputes between neighbours, missing persons or lost property

> (*Wilson and Ashton 1998*, p. 125)

Helping people to find a suitable plumber as part of the caring function carries nowhere near as much legitimacy as squads of dedicated officers doggedly pursuing criminals and the 'thin blue line' protecting life and liberty from marauders and rioters.

Many officers appear to believe, and sometimes publicly promote the idea, that chaos will descend unless the police hold it at bay. Thus, while the law enforcement and order maintenance aspects of the police role are obviously important and should not be underestimated, they enjoy a massive *symbolic* importance today beyond their actual operational incidence and effectiveness.

It was not always thus. As Chapter 2 highlighted, the post-war period up to the early 1960s was characterized by a peacekeeping approach in which there was no over-riding emphasis upon strict law enforcement. Furthermore, the need to restore order following major outbreaks of public unrest was rarely required. However, as Cain (1973) and Holdaway (1977) show, the peacekeeping style of policing gave way throughout the remainder of the 1960s and the early 1970s to a more aggressive form of law enforcement policing – namely, so-called 'fire-brigade policing' in which the major police response was to react to calls for assistance in crime matters. This change came about not only as a result of developments in society itself, but also, more crucially, as a result of the drive within the police for greater technological sophistication, and increased specialization and professionalization. These developments within the police, in turn, brought about a fundamental shift in police-public relations and led to greater social distance between the two. The generally high levels of trust, confidence and co-operation between the police and the public declined and, in some inner-city areas, were almost completely eroded. The everyday contact that the police enjoyed with the public on non-crime-related matters, and which had helped to create such trust were now to an important extent replaced by strictly crime-related relationships (Stephens 1988).

By the mid-1970s the police were increasingly portraying themselves as a *professional* organization with highly specialized skills and knowledge to bring to the fight against crime. As they had been unchallenged for so long, they had grown accustomed to viewing themselves as experts in fighting crime and as the only possible group of professionals able to take and implement *operational* decisions in the law enforcement and order maintenance spheres. Complementing this image of professionalism and expertise was the growing and often highly visible array of technological aids deployed by the police. The inner-city riots of the early and mid-1980s and the resulting swift development of the police's paramilitary tactics, training and equipment brought their order maintenance capabilities, like those of their law enforcement approach, into the modern era (Manwaring-White 1983). Cultivating an image of a force in control allowed the police to become more powerful. Nonetheless, in recent years, the police's confidence (and to some extent its power) has been dented by its general failure significantly to reduce crime and improve clear-up rates, by a series of corruption scandals and by persistent allegations of sexual and racial discrimination – developments that have helped make the police more willing to listen to the public and to adopt a less abrasive policing style. Even so, the perception remains very strong among many officers that the essential roles of the police are still those of law enforcement and order maintenance. In short, the police culture, especially the canteen culture, is still largely based on the idea of control, rather than service or care.

A CULTURE OF CONTROL

As mentioned in Chapter 2, the police force is not a monolithic organization and, accordingly, there is no single police culture. For example, senior management's cultural understanding of the role of the police will not be identical to those of sergeants and constables. However, all officers have an interest in control; more specifically in being *in control*. Unpredictability is perceived as potentially dangerous by officers, especially those at the 'sharp end' of policing on the streets. Being in control, therefore, lessens the chances of injury, of an operation going wrong, or of unwelcome and unintended consequences arising. Public order events where the police may adopt a clear paramilitary approach and dress in paramilitary clothing, and law enforcement or crime control operations such as stop and search, intelligence-led policing and zero tolerance are all good examples of the culture of control being put into practice.

Public order and paramilitarism

It is in *restoring* order when disorder has broken out that the police's paramilitary role is most in evidence. In recent years the two most notable examples of this role were the police's involvement in urban riots such as in Brixton (and elsewhere) in 1981, and in the national miners' strike in 1984–1985.

The Brixton riots in April 1981 were a public demonstration that the use of hard-line policing tactics, such as stop and search, in racially sensitive areas can have most unfortunate and unintended consequences. The intensive activities in the area that were part of a police operation known as 'Swamp 81' (during which many black people were stopped by the police) helped to spark off some of the worst rioting known in mainland Britain. Immediately following the disturbances, the government appointed a High Court judge, Lord Scarman, to investigate the riots and their causes. He concluded that the violence associated with the disorder was a 'spontaneous reaction of the crowds to what they believed to be police harassment'. Moreover, the riots 'were essentially an outburst of anger and resentment by young black people against the police' (Scarman 1981, p. 45). This combination of potentially destructive law enforcement by the police and distinct racism was re-enacted in UK cities throughout the 1980s to the detriment of police-public relations, especially those with ethnic minorities.

The Brixton riots and other disturbances that summer, and the 1981 Scarman Report itself, were watersheds in the style of policing. Keen to improve police-public relations, Scarman included a host of recommendations to update police training so that it could better cope with a multi-racial society. He argued for better probationer training for recruits, greater emphasis on community relations and the development of race-awareness training. However, although the police made some progress in all three fields throughout the 1980s, the least successful area was that related to race-awareness training (Home Office 1983). Scarman also recommended training in public order techniques, such as the use of shields for the lower ranks, and instruction in tactics and strategies to handle disorder for senior police officers. It was *this* area of police training, rather than those related to communication skills and police-public relations, that took off after 1981.

The Brixton and other riots led the police to believe that they were poorly equipped and trained to handle such massive outbreaks of public disorder. A difficult line had to be trodden between ensuring that the police were adequately protected against injury during times of disorder (and thus able to protect the lives and property of citizens) while not giving the police a free hand to quell disorder as brutally as they might like, and with no concern for appropriate behaviour. Not surprisingly, the police accorded a very high priority to paramilitary training, especially after 1981. As one chief constable of the period stated:

8970

> Training now takes account of our experiences of 1981, and has been formulated at national level. All police officers who might be called to police outbreaks of disorder are now trained in the techniques of the use of riot shields singly and in groups and formations. They are instructed in the new tactics designed to remove the initiative from rioters and give the police service a much more flexible approach ...
>
> (Oxford 1984, p. 123)

The *national* development of paramilitary training common to all officers and police forces, coupled with the implementation of new paramilitary tactics (kept secret from the public), greatly enhanced the police's public order capabilities. Their new power, and the effectiveness of their new training and tactics, were put to use only a few years later in the miners' strike. Whether this 12-month struggle between police and pickets amounted to a more 'flexible approach' or constituted a grave abuse of civil liberties is still being debated.

The miners' strike of 1984–1985 was a turning point in this country, not only for industrial relations, but also in the use of paramilitary policing. Looked at from one point of view, the police were protecting the rights of non-striking miners to go into work unmolested by the pickets outside the collieries; looked at from another, the government were abusing the independence of the police and using them to break an industrial dispute. Some police officers themselves wondered whether they were being used to preserve law and order or to implement government policy (Scraton 1985, p. 159). During the strike the police were seen to engage in a variety of tactics that earned them trenchant criticism from some academic quarters and deep-seated dislike from some sections of the public – not least in the striking coal-mining areas (NCCL 1984; McIlroy 1985). In particular, the police were accused of moving too quickly from containing the situation to assaulting pickets in an indiscriminate manner (McIlroy 1985, p. 107).

The tactics deployed (including the use of horses) were dictated by a confidential manual, *Public Order Tactical Operations*, that had been compiled following the 1980–1981 riots by the Association of Chief Police Officers (ACPO) with help from police officers from Northern Ireland and Hong Kong with their traditions of 'colonial-style' policing. (Such a style placed much greater emphasis on the use of paramilitary force against civilian populations.) Moreover, because of the national dimension of paramilitary training, ACPO rank officers could now order any tactic from the manual to be carried out safe in the knowledge that everyone under their command would be able to implement the order. Another disturbing national element in the whole strike was the National Reporting Centre based in London and headed by an ACPO member. Because of the scale and length of the strike and its particular geographical distribution, individual police forces could not cope with the public order demands made on them. In such circumstances the police can agree to provide mutual aid so that officers from the Metropolitan Police, for example, could be sent to help their colleagues in Nottinghamshire and Yorkshire where the picketing was frequently at its most intense. The whole process of co-ordinating and implementing this system of mutual aid was operated from the National Reporting Centre, which during the period of the strike became, de facto, the headquarters of a *single*, *centralized* and *national* police force, in complete contrast to the tradition of local police constabularies under some semblance of local control.

The miners' strike tells us much about the power of the state and the role of the police during periods of extreme disturbances. The police's paramilitary role is now essentially a national capability, but one that is, arguably, largely unaccountable to the public. Furthermore, the police continue to learn lessons from their paramilitary experiences so that their preparedness for conflict is regularly enhanced. For instance, following widespread rioting at Broadwater Farm in 1985 and the death of a police officer, the Metropolitan Police instigated a review of its public order capabilities, and, in more recent years, the police as a whole have been at the forefront in lobbying government about the use of new technologies, such as CS gas sprays for individual officers to carry.

During the 1990s the police have not been faced with a strike like that of the miners nor riots like Brixton and Broadwater Farm. Their paramilitary capability has not, however, vanished. Nor should we assume that during some future conflict we will not see the same mistakes being made, in which police containment of a group of people too easily and quickly escalates into police aggression and unacceptable methods with which to impose their control. Fortunately, better planning and preparation is being put in place for public events where there is the potential for disorder – in order to ensure that officers do not lose control and, therefore, do not themselves have to employ violent paramilitary tactics. Waddington's study of the Metropolitan

Police is a good example of this development.

During his period of research on the Metropolitan Police, Waddington (1994) was intrigued that the police do not make more extensive use of their paramilitary powers under the Public Order Act 1986. According to him, the police prefer to minimize trouble and to avoid confrontation at all costs in order to remain in control of events. Confrontation with the public at a march or rally might very well lead to trouble for officers; on-the-job trouble would flow from having to deploy their paramilitary capabilities, and in-the-job trouble would entail internal enquiries into what went wrong and possibly severe criticism from public and politicians (Waddington 1994, pp. 40–2). It is considered far better, therefore, to avoid both kinds of trouble by ensuring that the passage of events always remains under police control. The main way in which the police ensure their control over marches and demonstrations is through negotiation with event organizers. Control is further enhanced by the police gathering prior information on the nature of the people likely to be involved in the event. In addition, extensive planning and preparation goes into the manner in which the event is to be policed and, most importantly, the police exercise control over the area where the event is to take place or over which route it will pass – the 'ground'. The police feel that they 'own' this ground, and police-controlled ground usually presents few problems for the police. It is when the police are about to *lose* control over events or over the ground that they are most likely to intervene in a paramilitary fashion and, thus, to run the risk of widespread confrontation.

Stop and search

The Police and Criminal Evidence Act (PACE) 1984 gave the police wide-ranging powers to stop and search people and vehicles, provided they had reasonable grounds for suspicion. Stop and search activities usually arise when officers, some in plain clothes, concentrate their efforts in a particular locality in an attempt to reduce levels of crime. Stop and search operations must be handled with great sensitivity (especially in areas with high proportions of ethnic minorities) for they have a strong potential to undermine police-public relations and to be perceived as a form of police harassment. Although stop and search powers are widely used by the police, there is continuing debate about the definition of 'reasonable suspicion' and whether in fact the police are acting lawfully (Brown, D. 1997). Use of stop and search and the percentage of arrests stemming from them vary greatly between police forces, with the Metropolitan Police making most use of these powers. For instance, in 1995 Cleveland Constabulary carried out 12,539 searches under PACE powers, leading to 910 arrests or 7.3% of arrests as a proportion of PACE searches. West Mercia had a similar number of searches but a higher arrest rate; the figures were 12,024 searches and 1,909 arrests (15.9%). Surrey and Greater Manchester constabularies had similar percentage arrest rates (12.3% and 11.6%), but searched widely different numbers – respectively 14,878 and 49,234 individuals (Home Office 1997e, p. 72). In 1997–1998 the Metropolitan Police searched 336,692 people, of whom it arrested 37,624 (11.2%).

It is not known how many of these arrests result in actual criminal *convictions*, but a hit rate among English and Welsh forces ranging from one in six to more than one in ten people being arrested after a search would not, on the face of it, indicate particular success.

> Looking at the 'success' of searches in terms of the proportion producing arrests, effectiveness has gradually declined: currently, one in eight results in arrest. Around two-thirds of those arrested are eventually charged or cautioned
>
> (Brown, D. 1997, p. 2)

Indeed, since 1997 the position has deteriorated. In 1998 a record number of people were stopped and searched by the police in England and Wales. Of the 1,050,700 people who were stopped – a 20% increase on the year before – only one in ten stops led to an arrest, the lowest proportion overall since 1986 when PACE powers of stop and search came into being.

The Metropolitan Police justify their stop and search policy by arguing that it helps to catch criminals and deters others from committing offences, all of which adds up to fewer victims of crime and greater public safety. Against these benefits must be weighed the damage to race relations in particular that such activities may be causing (to which subject we return later in this chapter). Stop and search operations may play a part in fighting crime, but their worth should not be exaggerated. Furthermore, unless people are treated with care and sensitivity when stopped, such exercises have the very real potential for souring police-public relations. In cultural terms, what stop and search operations signify is the police's concern to exercise control over an area by filling it with officers whose sole purpose is to stop and search 'likely looking' individuals, most of whom are law-abiding citizens going about their lawful business.

Intelligence-led policing

Since 'traditional' policing methods have not been significantly successful in beating crime, intelligence-led policing was introduced as a new approach concentrating on finding acceptable evidence against serious or repeat offenders (Davies *et al.* 1998, p. 401). It has three facets. First, there is the police's surveillance capacity, which allows them to target criminals who may operate across force boundaries. Second, there are specialist squads that target criminals who may operate across basic command units or divisions within individual forces. Third, each basic command unit or division may have its own proactive teams or a group of CID officers who will target the activities of local criminals, such as prolific burglars (Audit Commission 1993, p. 57). Intelligence-led policing is a more proactive style of policing, which requires greater teamwork, a keener focus on the more serious (or frequent) crimes, and greater use of informants. Two major examples of such an approach have been Metropolitan Police initiatives code-named Operation Bumblebee and Operation Eagle Eye, both set up in recent years.

Operation Bumblebee is the largest anti-burglary initiative in England and Wales and has the aim of arresting burglars and deterring would-be burglars. Through targeting known repeat-offenders and staging raids on their homes, the operation has been credited with bringing about a dramatic decrease in the rate of burglary in London and in improving the clear-up figures. Operation Eagle Eye targets muggers in response to growing fears among Londoners concerning street crime. As with Operation Bumblebee, the anti-mugging initiative uses a combination of intelligence, surveillance and targeting of suspects to combat this problem. Previously such methods would only have been deployed in connection with the most serious crimes but now they are being used in a specific and targeted manner. The Metropolitan Police have introduced new technology as part of Operation Eagle Eye and have run a high-profile publicity campaign to indicate to muggers that the police are determined to catch them, and to the public that one of its major concerns is being addressed. Many of the Metropolitan Police's divisions have been equipped with new surveillance cameras and computerized witness albums as well as extensive computer software to help them track and analyse the movements of muggers – a small number of whom are responsible for the majority of such crimes.

During its first year of operation in 1995 the number of recorded street robberies in London remained static, compared with a 26% increase for the year before. However, figures for 1996 and 1997 indicated a fall of 5% in street robberies and an improvement in clear-up rates. While further research needs to be done before the full worth of activities such as Operation Eagle Eye can be analysed, there have been, nevertheless, some improvements in the overall situation, which have been attributed to the following characteristics of intelligence-led initiatives.

- Police effort, resources and technology are focused on a clear and strong strategy.
- There is a greater emphasis on proactivity, use of intelligence and crime-pattern analysis to indicate where to focus resources.
- There is an increased emphasis on bringing about crime reduction through partnerships with the public and other agencies (Stockdale and Gresham 1998).

Zero tolerance

This style of policing came from America, especially New York whose mayor, Rudolph Giuliani, and former Chief of Police, William J. Bratton, are keen supporters. At first sight it appears to offer all sorts of advantages for cracking down on crime but, although it has been much discussed in the UK, it has only been put into limited practice in a few areas, such as Hartlepool. Essentially, zero tolerance draws on the 'broken window' philosophy, which suggests that small signs of social decay and disorder, such as broken windows, may encourage more serious crimes to be committed because there is a sense that no one cares about the particular area any longer. Accordingly, *all* forms of anti-social behaviour in a specific locality must be tackled by the police and prevented, for otherwise this behaviour will lead to more serious crimes and to a greater deterioration in the quality of the lives of the people living in that area. Support for the zero tolerance approach is based on the British Crime Survey findings that disorderly neighbourhoods and higher crime-rates are associated; indeed, Jack Straw, the Home Secretary, has indicated that zero tolerance (in a broader form than just policing) will play an integral part in the government's plans to tackle disorder and incivility.

In its policing format, supporters of zero tolerance tend to be sensitive about its nomenclature. Dennis (1998), for example, argued that zero tolerance is not about intolerance but about confidence – confident policing should be as tolerant as possible but also completely clear that its goal is to prevent anti-social behaviour. Zero tolerance policing is based on three major ideas.

- Nipping things in the bud prevents anti-social groups from believing that their members are in charge of a locality and, thereby, stops them from gravitating towards more serious offences.
- Police officers should deploy 'low-intensity, humane, good-natured control' when confronted by relatively minor anti-social activities.
- By building on the first two ideas of tolerant control to reduce petty crime, vandalism and low-level disorder, a locality will become less attractive to more serious criminals (Dennis 1998, p. 3).

Clearly, such an approach fits in well with the police's cultural need to be in control of events (Dennis and Mallon 1998, p. 63). However, not all police officers are supporters of zero tolerance. For example, Chief Constable Pollard of the Thames Valley Police was concerned that zero tolerance was too simplistic an approach (Pollard 1998). Policing in England and Wales is now more partnership oriented and such partnerships are needed if disorderly and run-down localities are to be transformed – because social problems cannot be tackled by policing alone. Moreover, many of the activities that zero tolerance would crack down on are not illegal (though they may certainly be annoying or worse), and this raises issues about civil liberties. If the police were routinely to deploy heavy-handed tactics in trying to stamp out anti-social and minor illegal activities, they could soon lose the respect and co-operation of the public. Any short-term gains from a zero tolerance approach would then be lost and longer-term problems could arise as the public withdrew their support for the police. In the worst case, if police tactics were especially uncompromising, civil disorder might ensue (Pollard 1998).

Zero tolerance is a reflection of the generally punitive mood that has gripped America in recent years, but finding scape goats for the crime problem and targetting citizens in an aggressive manner is unlikely to be the answer to this particular social problem. Research suggests that zero tolerance can lead to overzealous policing, which is damaging to police-public relations (Home Office 1996a, pp. 72–3).

Control, machismo and territoriality

Another important aspect of the police culture of control is the police's sense of territoriality. For example, territoriality was an important factor in the way in which the miners' strike was policed, just as today it is a factor in the many other kinds of law enforcement and order maintenance operations that the police mount. The police are not just offended (as might be expected) by criminals committing crimes and causing them embarrassment, they also take umbrage against anyone who violates their 'ground', as Waddington's (1994) research has already illustrated. The idea that the police 'own' and control the areas for which they are responsible is nowhere better set out than by Holdaway (1984, p. 36) who argued that despite many indications to the contrary, the police hold strongly to the notion that all territory is 'police-controlled territory'. It is as if any attempt to undermine this control is a threat to the predominantly male-dominated and 'macho' culture of the lower ranks, and any such threat runs the risk of a brusque and, at times, brutal response.

Clearly, control does not necessarily have to be implemented through the use of aggressive tactics. Indeed, good communication and social skills are vital to tolerant policing, and many officers have such skills and are keen to deploy them. Research suggests that female officers are 'less aggressive, better able to manage violent confrontations, and more pleasant and respectful to citizens' (Brown, J. 1997, p. 37).

The canteen culture will be difficult to eradicate, but it can be diluted by the introduction into the police of more women and ethnic minorities, and more recruits with a higher level of educational attainment. This could help achieve a better balance of personnel within the police force – a balance that will better serve the ethic of a caring police organization and be more representative of the population at large.

CONTROL AND POLICE CULTURE: POTENTIAL DANGERS

Clearly, the police need certain powers and must be able to exercise a certain level of control if they are to carry out their duties effectively. Equally clear is the need for police powers to be subject to checks and balances; and the police should be accountable to the public. It is all a question of maintaining a balance between fighting crime and maintaining order and the individual rights of citizens; between the power of the state, mediated through the police, and the protection of due process. A police force that is too powerful and insufficiently accountable, that places too much emphasis on strategies of control and that has at its heart a bloody-minded and often unbending canteen culture, can too easily adopt practices that alienate significant sections of the public. The potential for the abuse of police powers and for growing public disenchantment exists in areas such as the use of technology and its possible threat to civil liberties, and in the disturbing evidence of police corruption. As discussed earlier, one particular area in which police power is often used in a damaging way is that of race.

Stereotyping and race

We all use stereotypes to some extent; I for one will never be convinced that Arsenal are anything other than boring! However, when police officers do so there is a danger that their power and discretion will be used in a discriminatory manner. It is still the case that too many officers stereotype black people as criminals (Smith and Gray 1985, p. 406). For example, Holdaway (1996, p. 9) found that many officers consistently assumed that black people committed violent crime. Furthermore, a large-scale study of the Metropolitan Police in the early 1980s reported that racist language and racial prejudice were commonplace among many police officers (Smith and Gray 1985, p. 388). Of course, it is possible to hold racist attitudes without acting on them, but the evidence suggests that ethnic minorities do frequently experience prejudice and discrimination from the police. Worse still, when ethnic minorities become victims of racially motivated crime, the frequent complaint is that the police do not take the matter seriously. Furthermore, there is wide variation between police forces concerning the information that they collect on racial incidents. In a classic 'double-bind' situation, 'people from ethnic minorities are simultaneously over-policed by their local police force and under-serviced by them when they find themselves to be the victims of crime…' (Walklate 1996, p. 200). In the early 1990s, Afro-Caribbeans were nearly four times more likely than white people to be stopped on foot by the police (Southgate and

Crisp 1992). A later Home Office (1997e) evaluation confirmed earlier findings that black people figure disproportionately in arrests relative to whites. Some of the latest research has found that Afro-Caribbeans were more likely than any other ethnic group to be stopped on foot or in a car by the police, and were more prone to multiple stops. In addition, they were more than twice as likely as white people to be searched when stopped by the police and four times more likely to be arrested (Bucke 1997, p. 1). Such apparent 'targeting' of certain sections of the public cannot but reflect badly on the police.

CONCLUSION

This chapter has been rather harsh on the police because of its focus on issues of control, where the potential for abuse of police powers is greatest. That is not to deny that the same potential exists in some of the caring aspects of the police role. For example, some critics (Scraton 1985) see extensive inter-agency co-ordination to prevent crime as an insidious form of police-led 'soft control' with its own threats to civil liberties. However, whether predominantly caring or controlling, police activities must be accountable. Moreover, the police also need to work harder to improve the quality and diversity of their recruits, to train them more effectively and, through modern management practices, to begin to stamp out the worst excesses of the canteen culture. In this way they may avoid the repetition of the types of events detailed in this chapter. Although they have made good progress in some of these organizational areas (for which they should be commended) the task is not finished. Indeed, some might argue that the task of maintaining a proper balance between the power of the police and the rights of citizens is one that can never be finished.

KEY POINTS

- The police place great cultural value on their order maintenance and crime control duties.
- Officers have both a cultural and a personal interest in being in control of events.
- Threats to the police's perceptions of control, especially control over police 'ground' or territory, are likely to escalate into disorder.

- Stop and search activities, intelligence-led policing and zero tolerance policing are all examples of police controlling activities.
- Ethnic minorities, by virtue of police racism, are frequently the 'victims' of these controlling activities.
- More female and ethnic minority officers in the police would help to combat cultural stereotypes held by the members of the canteen culture, and improve police-public relations.

GUIDE TO FURTHER READING

There is a highly informative account of race relations within the police and between the police and the public, and of policy responses to racism in Holdaway, S. (1996) *The Racialisation of British Policing*, London: Macmillan. There are also good sections on stereotyping, and the police occupational culture and the place of racism within it.

There is a compelling critique of zero tolerance policing in Bratton, W., Dennis, N. (ed.), Griffiths, W., Mallon, R., Orr, J. and Pollard, C. (1998) *Zero Tolerance. Policing a Free Society*, London: Institute of Economic Affairs, 2nd edition.

In Francis, P., Davies, P. and Jupp, V. (eds) (1997) *Policing Futures. The Police, Law Enforcement and the Twenty-First Century*, Basingstoke: Macmillan, a variety of writers make contributions on equal opportunities and the police, controlling crime, providing a service, managerial challenges facing the police, and even on policing the Internet.

For wide-ranging and informative coverage on policing, including public order policing and the use of 'deadly force', see Leishman, F., Loveday, B. and Savage, S. (eds) (1996) *Core Issues in Policing*, London: Longman.

An overview of the criminal justice system

4

Outline
- Separate criminal justice systems exist in Northern Ireland and in Scotland; this chapter deals only with the system in England and Wales.
- The system is under great pressure to process large numbers of cases and to do so in a fair and just manner, according to the ideals of due process.
- The major components of the system are the police, the adult and youth courts, the probation service, the Crown Prosecution Service and the prisons.

THE WORK AND GOALS OF THE CRIMINAL JUSTICE SYSTEM

The criminal justice system in England and Wales is under enormous pressure and must respond to huge demands daily. The extent of its workload and costs is illustrated in Table 4.1. The statistics in this table actually represent a period when recorded crime was falling. Since then, some of these figures have worsened; and although crime has continued to fall there has been no appreciable improvement in the overall clear-up rate. The prison population has also increased dramatically from its 1996 figure. (The reasons for the latter seeming paradox are explained later when we look at sentencing trends.)

Table 4.1 Criminal Justice in England and Wales – some selected statistics for 1996

	(to nearest thousand)
Notifiable offences recorded by the police	5,036,000
Proportion of notifiable offences cleared up	27%
Proceedings in Magistrates' Courts	1,930,000
Trials in Crown Courts	90,000
Persons convicted or cautioned	1,734,000
Persons supervised by the Probation Service	169,000
Daily average prison population	55,000
Police officers employed	127,000
Prison staff employed	38,000
Total costs: £10,000 million per year and rising	

Source: Home Office 1997a

In addition to trying to stem increases in crime and to provide the best value for money, all modern systems of criminal justice attempt to achieve four major goals:

- the conviction of those guilty of crimes
- the acquittal of those who are innocent
- the protection of the general public from crime
- the provision of some form of restitution to the victims of crime.

DUE PROCESS

The first two goals relate most closely to the courts, where a balance has to be struck between the powers of the prosecution and the rights of the defence in order for a fair system to prevail. Under the notions of 'due process' that operate in the system of justice in England and Wales people are presumed innocent of any charge unless they are found guilty in a court of law, or admit their guilt in order to receive a police caution. They are also entitled to legal representation.

A production line for making cars is referred to as a continuous assembly system, often involving a good deal of automation. Such a system is considered the most efficient way of making a highly complicated machine. Although the criminal justice system is also complicated, it would not dare adopt the equivalent of a continuous assembly system for to do so would mean that the innocent risked being wrongly convicted as they were swept along on a tide of efficiency. If efficiency were all that we cared about in criminal justice in this country then we would not apply standards to it, such as those applying to the questioning of people detained by the police, nor would we permit cumbersome jury deliberations, nor ensure the existence of various procedural safeguards. Fortunately, justice is about more than efficiency; it is about openness and fairness and protecting the rights of those who become caught up in the system but who may well be innocent. Thus, if an analogy is to be used, the criminal justice system is better seen as an obstacle course, in which a series of impediments must be overcome before someone can be convicted of a crime. One of these obstacles is the need to gather and present evidence in procedurally acceptable ways. Furthermore, the courts must not only protect the procedural and other rights of all defendants, but also must not discriminate on the basis of defendants' race, religion, class or gender. This protection of due process procedures is central to the working of the system, and is an important way in which the system remains just towards those suspected of crime.

It is the police who are primarily concerned with the third goal; namely, protecting the public from crime. However, when crime occurs, the police, the courts and other organizations within the criminal justice system are all responsible for investigating and processing these incidences of wrong-doing. In this sense, citizens are not left powerless in the face of crime because they can look to the law for resolution. Of course, no system can protect it citizens perfectly, and no system solves all crime or resolves all of the problems presented by criminality. Moreover, democratic societies do not give unfettered power to their criminal justice agencies but ensure that there are proper curbs on them. Thus, the police must have reasonable suspicion in order to arrest someone; they cannot deprive people of their liberty on a whim. The Crown Prosecution Service must have sufficient evidence to proceed; it cannot take a case forward on the basis of malice but must act on what proof it has that a person committed a crime. However, although these particular safeguards help to minimize the number of innocent people who are wrongly convicted, the principles of justice and fairness do not end there. So, for instance, the prisons should not subject inmates to brutality and ill-treatment; prisoners still have certain rights and must not be treated in an inhuman fashion. All of these examples demonstrate the way in which the criminal justice system is supposed to act fairly and to balance the need to protect the public while detecting and punishing the wrong-doers. However, as the following chapters will highlight – and as you will already have understood from the chapters on the police – the system does not always live up to these ideals. One particular example of its failure to do so relates to the fourth goal – having regard to the needs of victims – which is one that has only recently been given prominence within the criminal justice system. Many would argue that victims are still not well served by the system and that much more needs to be done to help and support them (Gibson and Cavadino 1995, pp. 154–60).

In recognition of this, the government proposed in late 1998 to introduce legislation that would restrict details of a person's previous sexual history being divulged in trials involving rape and serious sexual offences. Moreover, more attention is to be given to the needs of witnesses (many of whom are also victims) through plans to provide new rights to appear in court to severely disabled witnesses. Vulnerable witnesses will also be allowed to give their evidence behind screens, or by using video-recorded interviews and live television links in courtrooms, and knowledge of the identity of witnesses in some more sensitive cases will be restricted. Furthermore, more and more governmental bodies and criminal justice agencies are having to take greater account of the needs and rights of victims.

SYSTEM COMPONENTS

Like all systems, the criminal justice system is composed of a number of essential elements not all of which are as closely interrelated or co-ordinated as one might suppose (Gibson and Cavadino 1995, p. 10). Indeed, political responsibility for the components is divided among various government departments, with the Home Office overseeing the police, probation and prison services, and the criminal law. The Lord Chancellor's Department covers the Magistrates' and Crown Courts, while the Crown Prosecution Service is accountable to the Attorney General. Even so, it is possible to trace the typical route of those entering the system and to put further detail on the work of its major agencies. Depending on their age, the severity of the offence, and other relevant factors, it is quite simple to trace a person's progress through the system.

The police and the Crown Prosecution Service

The vast majority of cases that enter the criminal justice system begin with the police. The police are responsible for investigating crime, maintaining (or restoring) public order, and arresting and charging those suspected of having committed crimes. As discussed earlier, they also have a crime prevention function and a facilitating role in victim support (Stephens and Becker 1994). In the case of minor crimes where the person admits guilt, the police frequently decide that an official warning (formerly a caution) will suffice. Offences not deemed suitable for this option are investigated by the police and the evidence they gather is forwarded to the Crown Prosecution Service (CPS). Since 1986 it has been the responsibility of the CPS to decide whether to prosecute or to discontinue a case (either because it is thought that the evidence is not sufficient to provide a realistic prospect of a conviction, or because it is deemed not to be in the public interest to proceed). For instance, there may be ample evidence against an individual to secure a conviction, but the personal circumstances of that person may be such – terminal illness, to cite one example – that the CPS decides a prosecution would not be in the public interest (Davies *et al.* 1995).

The criminal courts

If the CPS decides to prosecute, then the defendant will appear before one of three courts. When a child (between the ages of 10 and 17) is accused of a crime, other than the most serious, that child will appear before the Youth Court. However, most child offenders receive a police caution for relatively trivial offences, and an appearance in the Youth Court is generally reserved for weightier matters. Those aged 18 years and above appear in the Magistrates' Court for relatively minor or summary offences (such as minor criminal damage), or in the Crown Court for serious or indictable acts (such as robbery). All three types of court are distributed throughout the towns and cities of England and Wales. Indeed, the *local* administration and operation of justice, albeit under central policy direction, is a feature of the system. Magistrates' Courts are presided over either by a single legally qualified and salaried stipendiary magistrate, or (more frequently) by a panel of three lay magistrates who are essentially public-spirited volunteers known as JPs or Justices of the Peace. They are not legally qualified but have received some training, and are paid only expenses. Typically, accused individuals are defended by a professionally qualified solicitor who may be paid for out of the Legal Aid scheme, which is provided to help those who are too poor to pay for their own lawyer (Gibson and Cavadino 1995).

In late 1998 the government indicated that it would massively overhaul the system of legal representation for defendants as part of its Access to Justice Bill. Criminal Legal Aid is to be abolished and replaced by a Criminal Defence Service (CDS), which will award contracts to lawyers to carry out public-funded representation in criminal cases. The CDS is intended to cut the waste and bureaucracy in the Legal Aid system, which in 1998 cost £733 million to run. The contracts will be for fixed-price service, agreed in advance with legal providers so as to encourage lawyers to reduce delays and to work more efficiently. Lawyers employed directly by the CDS – similar to the public-defender figures familiar in the USA – will defend a small number of cases, but most will still be handled by lawyers in private practice. However, the Law Society, which represents lawyers in private practice, fears that campaigning lawyers (whom the government may see as 'troublemakers') could be excluded from the new system of contracts. In addition, the proposed changes are clearly intended to reduce costs and to increase government control. This runs the risk that what will emerge will be a culture of uncontested, plea-bargained cases, which lets the guilty off too lightly and punishes the innocent for something they haven't done but which they may have been pressurized into falsely admitting. (Plea-bargaining refers to a situation where a defendant pleads guilty to a lesser charge in exchange for more serious charges being dropped or in anticipation of a more lenient sentence.)

In the Crown Court a judge presides over cases, ensures fair play and provides a summation and appropriate guidance for the jury at the end of the trial. A Crown Court judge is typically a former barrister of some repute or 'Queen's Counsel', the term given to senior advocates. It is the jury composed of twelve randomly selected members of the public, in secret deliberation, that decides on the guilt or otherwise of the defendant. Trying to provide reasons why the jury should acquit the defendant is the task of the defence barrister, who is instructed by the defence solicitor – both of whom may be paid out of public funds. The Crown Court is much more formal than the Magistrates' Court and in the former the judge and prosecuting and defending barristers all wear wigs and gowns.

Magistrates' Courts dispense 'quick' or summary justice without the need for a jury, and about 96% of all criminal cases are handled here. Often, defendants don't even have to attend court but can plead guilty by letter, for instance, to a range of motoring offences. Some criminal offences can be tried in either the Magistrates' or the Crown Courts and in these cases it is for the defendant (with the advice of the defence counsel) to decide which to opt for. In general, more severe sentences are handed down in the Crown Court where the more serious cases are heard, but there is also provision for someone found guilty in the Magistrates' Court to be referred to the Crown Court for sentencing where the lower court feels that the deserved sentence is beyond its own powers to impose (Barclay 1995).

In May 1999 the government proposed to abolish trial by jury for a range of offences, which would affect around 22,000 people per year. Those accused of 'either-way' offences such as minor theft and indecent assault would no longer be able automatically to opt for trial by jury. The government argued that such a change would prevent the 18,500 cases in 1998 in which defendants abused the system and caused further delays and costs by opting for the Crown Court only then to change their pleas to guilty just before the actual trial. Critics countered that the proposals would add to costs since more people would appeal against the refusal of a jury trial by JPs and that trying such cases only before magistrates would lead to still more miscarriages of justice.

While the two adult courts are normally open to members of the public who can watch proceedings from the public gallery, the public are not admitted to the Youth Court. Moreover, although the press may attend, they are rarely allowed to divulge the identities of the juvenile defendants and their families. Defendants in the Youth Court are children and, therefore, special efforts are made to protect their interests. The JPs who sit here are specially trained and have to take into account not only the demands of justice but also the needs of the defendant. This is the system of 'individualized' justice. In very simple terms, the adult courts operate a system of classical justice – one which is primarily concerned with the proper punishment of the wrong-doer and under which the courts are usually required to impose a penalty that is in keeping with the seriousness of the offence: the idea of 'just deserts'. However, in a Youth Court classical justice must be tempered with concern for the child's welfare. Hence, the focus on the individual circumstances of the child and family and the need to take into account what can be done not only to punish the delinquent, but also to 'treat' the delinquency so that the child turns away from committing further crime. The co-existence of punishment and welfare has not always worked well within the Youth Court (Stockdale and Casale 1992).

SENTENCING CONSIDERATIONS

In all three courts a defendant may be found not guilty or the case may be dropped for a number of reasons. In this scenario, the accused exits the criminal justice system a free person. However, if a defendant is found (or pleads) guilty, he or she is subject to a variety of sentences, depending on age, severity of the offence, previous criminal record, and so on. The court may call for a pre-sentence report before deciding on its sentence. (These are prepared by the probation service or social services for child offenders and concentrate on the offender's personal, family and educational background.) Some typical outcomes are an absolute or conditional discharge, or a fine, which are generally seen as 'light' sentences or punishments – low down on the tariff. Much higher on the tariff is imprisonment.

Custody

A defendant found guilty of a serious offence may well be sentenced to a period of incarceration in one of a variety of forms of custody that are age specific. Children aged 12 to 14 years old may be sent to a secure training centre. Teenagers and young offenders aged 15 to 20 may be sentenced to a period at a young offender institution, while adults may be imprisoned. Adult prisoners are allocated to one of the following kinds of prison: a high security or 'dispersal' prison for the most violent and dangerous inmates, a training or local prison, an open prison for those that can be reasonably trusted to serve their sentences in settings with the minimum of security, or a remand centre. There are 135 such institutions (as at August 1999) administered by the Prison Service, which is an executive agency of the Home Office. A small number of prisons are now run by the private sector. Prisons are essentially about two, often conflicting, goals – punishment and rehabilitation. Offenders are deprived of their liberty as a punishment, but many critics have argued that such has been the poor state of the prisons that incarceration has led to further punishment and humiliation being heaped on prisoners. In addition, some attempt is supposed to be made within prisons to turn offenders away from further crime – to reduce or eliminate recidivism – but it is argued that poor conditions, such as overcrowding, and too much emphasis on control and security militate against this goal (Blackstone 1990; Newburn 1995).

Community sentences

Another possible outcome for a convicted person is a community sentence – principally, probation, supervision, community service, and combination orders. These various orders are now regarded as penalties in their own right and no longer seen as alternatives to custody. They constitute what has been called 'punishment in the community' and, rather than being some kind of soft option, are supposed to ensure that offenders properly confront their offending behaviour and alter their criminal ways. It is the probation service, in the main, that is responsible for ensuring that this process takes place. There are 55 probation areas in England and Wales, employing 7,200 probation officers at the end of 1997 (which was the lowest December figure since 1991). It may be that government proposals to reorganize the service will mean that the number of probation areas is reduced to become coterminous with those of police forces in England and Wales. In addition to supervising those on community sentences, probation officers prepare pre-sentence reports for the courts and supervise prisoners, sentenced to more than 12 months, while in jail and after release. Over 600 probation officers work inside prisons, where they help prisoners to confront their offending behaviour and provide a link between their custodial experiences and subsequent supervision in the community (Stockdale and Casale 1992; Newburn 1995). Another form of community punishment is the curfew order, which is monitored by an electronic tag attached to the offender. (More detail is given on this and on community sentences in general in Chapter 8.)

In essence, these are the main routes for most offenders. At any stage in the process, a lack of evidence, or a serious breach of due process, may result in the suspected person leaving the system. Conversely, good evidence against someone will mean that they will remain within the system while its various officials decide how to proceed. Serious offences, especially those committed by adult males, tend to result in custodial sentences. With lesser offences, or where the courts have good reason not to incarcerate someone, there are a range of community sentences available.

Sentencing philosophy

Sentencers – magistrates and judges – must decide whether sentences will be primarily directed towards retribution, deterrence, protection of the public, rehabilitation of the offender, compensation or restitution to the victim or society in general, or a combination of these aims. The end product of sentencing decisions dictates, for instance, how many individuals receive community sentences and how many are sent to jail (and for how long). The decisions about sentencing aims taken in the courts in England and Wales, and the manner in which they are perceived, strongly influence the overall levels of satisfaction or criticism among the public, victims, police and other interested parties. In addition, there are standard sentencing principles, which are supposed to ensure that those sentenced are not treated unduly harshly and that there is a broad equity in sentencing across a range of offences and between different kinds of offenders (Harding and Koffman 1995). Thus, in deciding on a sentence a judge or magistrate will take into account:

- the circumstances and gravity of the offence in terms of value, consequences, or flagrant disregard for the law
- the degree of participation of the offender in the offence
- the extent to which the offender shows remorse for the offence
- the circumstances of the offender, such as previous criminal history, personal, family and employment (or school) background, and risk of re-offending
- the impact of the crime on the victim
- the plea in mitigation, which the defence lawyer provides to the court together with any details concerning the offender's reasons for committing the offence, and other matters considered to be favourable to the defendant's case

CONCLUSION

The criminal justice system is complicated, expensive to operate, frequently overwhelmed with cases, and confronted by many difficulties. Currently, there are three central issues that the system is struggling to resolve.

- What can be done to reduce the level of offending?
- What can be done for the victims of crime?
- What can be done with convicted offenders?

Each issue is problematic. In terms of reducing the levels of offending it may be that, in appropriate cases, bringing victim and criminal together so that the offender will appreciate at first hand the distress caused to the victim by the crime may lead to some reduction in further offences. But this does not indicate what one should do with convicted prisoners who have been sent to jail. Locking people up does not seem to bring about a drop in the rate of recidivism (Home Office 1998a, p. 131). In terms of what victims want, victims may not feel that jailing people is the most appropriate form of punishment and might want something more constructive to be done. In order both to help convicted offenders and to significantly reduce crime and its consequences, it may be necessary for institutions other than those of the criminal justice system (such as education and local authorities and employment agencies, to name a few) to play their part.

KEY POINTS

- All agencies within the criminal justice system work under tremendous caseload pressures.
- It is a very expensive system to maintain.
- At the heart of the system is the notion of due process.
- Typical criminals will probably follow the route of being investigated by the police, being prosecuted by the CPS, appearing in one of the criminal courts, being imprisoned, fined, or made subject to one of a variety of community penalties administered by the probation service.

GUIDE TO FURTHER READING

For a clear explanation of the nature of the criminal courts, due process, and the work of the police and the prison service, see Gibson, B. and Cavadino, P. (1995) *Introduction to the Criminal Justice Process*. Winchester: Waterside Press.

Useful chapters on the sentencing process, non-custodial sentences, and the prisons can be found in Harding, C. and Koffman, L. (1995) *Sentencing and the Penal System*, 2nd edition, London: Sweet and Maxwell.

There is detailed coverage of the role of the probation service and community penalties in Brownlee, I. (1998) *Community Punishment, A Critical Introduction*. London: Longman.

The youth question

5

Outline
- The youth justice system differs in important ways from the criminal justice system for adults because juveniles present special problems.
- Youth crime attracts particular public concern, sometimes bordering on moral panic.
- The history of youth justice policy has been characterized by a debate over the merits of the welfare versus the punishment approach to youth crime.
- The latest major attempt to redraw the lines of that debate was the Crime and Disorder Act 1998.

AN INTRODUCTION TO THE YOUTH JUSTICE SYSTEM

People aged 21 years and over are treated as adults by the criminal justice system and receive the penalties appropriate to their status. However, the youth justice system deals with those under the age of 21, and contains a range of penalties and options in keeping with those who have not yet fully matured. While young offender institutions provide custody for those aged between 15 and 20, the Youth Court only tries those between the ages of 10 and 17 years inclusively.

If someone between the ages of 10 and 17 is suspected of having committed a crime, the police must first decide what kind of action, if any, to take. They may decide to give the child an informal warning and leave it at that. However, if they are thinking of taking any kind of formal action, the police must interview the child in the presence of one parent or, failing that, an 'appropriate adult' (normally a social worker). Parent, appropriate adult or child may insist that a solicitor be present, who may be paid for out of Legal Aid funds. After the interview is completed, the police must decide on one of the following courses of formal action.

- The police will take no further action if they believe the child did not commit the offence.
- They may still take no further action if the offence was a very minor one.
- The police may issue a formal reprimand for first offenders (previously known as a 'caution') where the child admits the offence. The reprimand is normally administered by a senior police officer in the presence of the child's parent(s) and includes an admonishment about the child's future behaviour.
- For a subsequent offence the police may issue a warning – in which case a formal reprimand or caution is still given by a senior police officer at the police station, but in addition the child must submit to a plan designed to prevent further offending which is drawn up by a local youth offending team. The warning is similar to what used to be known as 'caution plus' schemes in which various kinds of short-term intervention focused on offending behaviour.
- The police may feel that the child should be prosecuted in the Youth Court in which case the file is forwarded to the Crown Prosecution Service for its decision.

When a young person is awaiting an appearance in the Youth Court, he or she is normally allowed home on police bail. However, the Youth Court itself may wish to set its own bail conditions where a young person is not living at home or, indeed, should not be permitted to live at home. Where the court sets conditional bail, the young person is normally allowed to live at home but has to abide by certain restrictions, such as being indoors at night. Many local areas have bail support schemes to help young people during this period when they are awaiting trial. If the court refuses bail, the young person may be looked after in a children's home or by foster parents, or remanded to a secure unit. In 1998 it was still possible to hold 15 and 16 year old boys on remand in prison, which was usually a special remand centre at a young offender institution. It is intended to phase out this practice as more secure accommodation becomes available.

THE YOUTH COURT: AN OUTLINE

The Youth Court, which came into being in October 1992 and replaced the Juvenile Court, deals with children (defined as being aged between 10 and 13 years inclusive) and with young persons (aged between 14 and 17 inclusive). Previously, the Juvenile Court did not deal with 17-year-olds, who had to be sent to the adult courts. In England and Wales the age of criminal responsibility begins at 10; it is higher in many other European countries. Where a child is charged with homicide, the case is tried in the Crown Court. There are also a small number of other circumstances where a child may be committed for trial in an adult court. The public are excluded from the Youth Court and although the proceedings may be reported in the press, the names of the young people are not normally divulged. Usually, three JPs sit in the court, and must include a man and a woman. The court has a range of sentences available, some of which depend on the age of the offender, including:

- an absolute or conditional discharge
- bind over of offender or parent
- a fine, for which a parent may be made responsible
- a compensation order, also for which a parent may be made responsible
- an attendance centre order
- a supervision order, which may also include specified restrictions, activities or residency requirements, and reparation
- a probation order for those aged 16 and above
- a community service order for those aged 16 and above
- a combination order for those aged 16 and above
- a curfew order for those aged 16 and above
- a reparation order requiring a young offender to make reparation to the victim or the community
- an action plan order in which the young offender must comply with an action plan to address offending behaviour
- a detention and training order, which is age specific, and requires a young offender to be subject to a period of custody followed by a period of supervision in the community. Secure training centres are available for persistent offenders aged between 12 and 14 years; those aged 15 and above may be sent to a young offender institution.

Further information on most of these sentences, and on other aspects of the Youth Court, can be found in Gibson and Cavadino (1995), and (for the sentences introduced by the Crime and Disorder Act 1998) in Audit Commission (1998a).

Youth Court magistrates receive special but limited training, which focuses on the differences between adult offending and criminal acts committed by juveniles, and it is the magistrates – rather than a jury – who decide guilt or innocence and who decide the sentence. Gibson and Cavadino (1995, p. 43) argue that the Youth Court represents one of the more enlightened aspects of criminal justice because of its duty to have regard for the welfare of the child. The welfare principle is not an overriding concern but must be balanced against the 'just deserts' philosophy contained in the Criminal Justice Act 1991. The major way in which the court arrives at decisions about the sentencing, and the welfare needs of the person, is through a pre-sentence report.

THE SCALE OF THE PROBLEM

The most serious outcome for a young offender is to be sentenced to a period of custody. Despite a 50% reduction between 1980 and 1992 in the number of young offenders aged 18 to 20 who were received into prison under sentence, the following years saw these numbers dramatically increase once more. Thus, in December 1997 there were 8,142 young offenders in prison under sentence (and a further 2,705 on remand), compared with 5,842 sentenced young people in June 1995, and a further 2,728 held on remand. Moreover, there has been a similar dramatic increase in the number of 15-year-olds being processed, convicted and sentenced by the Youth Court. The number of 15-year-olds found guilty by the courts rose from 8,162 in 1993 to 12,376 in 1995, an increase of 51.6%. Moreover, the courts have taken an increasingly punitive stance so that while 588 15-year-olds were sentenced directly to custody in 1993, this figure had risen to 874 in 1995. Shamefully, some 15-year-old boys and girls were still held in adult prisons – 267 of them were so accommodated on 7 March 1997. One reason for this increased punitiveness towards this age group is the relative decline in police cautions. Although the majority of 15-year-olds who commit an offence are still cautioned, the proportion has fallen. In 1993 the percentage of 15-year-olds cautioned was 86% for girls and 74% for boys. In 1995 these figures fell respectively to 79% and 62.5%, which meant that more children were being pushed into Youth Court appearances. This happened despite the fact that 70% of first-time 15-year-old offenders who receive a police caution do not re-offend. Against this, 89% of young males aged between 14 and 16 at sentencing were reconvicted of an offence within 2 years of being discharged from custody in 1992. This shows starkly the high rates of re-offending associated with custody, especially for young people.

A HISTORY OF YOUTH JUSTICE

Welfare versus punishment

Over the years there have been contrasting, and sometimes conflicting, approaches to juvenile offending. This may be summarized as the debate between welfare and punishment and, historically, youth justice policy has swung between these two principles. The welfare approach essentially tries to protect children from overzealous attention by the criminal justice system. It urges an appearance in the Youth Court only as a last resort and emphasizes the need to reduce the stigma and the potentially counter-productive effects of criminal prosecution, such as the high recidivism rates associated with custody. It preaches that society should have a certain 'tolerance' for what are, in the main, minor acts of delinquency and that society should seek to divert as many children as possible from the youth justice system in order to protect them from any undue harshness associated with trial and punishment. The welfare principle has also highlighted the possibility of the rehabilitation of young offenders through placing them in programmes that provide support, education and treatment.

Many of the proponents of the punishment approach, or the justice model, would argue that too great an emphasis on welfare leads to 'soft' measures, which fail not only to punish wrongdoers, but also to deter them from future acts. In the eighteenth century children were treated as if they were adults and could even be hanged. The nineteenth century saw a gradual reduction in this extremely punitive approach as legislators and policymakers became convinced that young people could be rehabilitated. The swing towards a greater emphasis on rehabilitation was helped by the rise of the medical profession with its focus on treatment, and by the increasing influence of social workers who stressed the value of working closely with offenders. Reflecting a more enlightened approach towards young offenders, a separate Juvenile Court was created in 1908. Since then the youth justice system has been characterized by a mixture of welfare and punishment philosophies.

Legislation and youth justice policy

However, at different times that mixture of philosophical approaches has varied. Another fillip for welfare adherents came with the Children and Young Persons Act 1933 with its stress on the need for courts to take into account the welfare of young people. But arguably the high point for the welfare approach was the Children and Young Persons Act 1969, which was 'based on a mixture of welfare and diversionary policies ...' (Davies *et al.* 1995, p. 137). Indeed, Worrall (1997, p. 129) describes the Act as 'the culmination of the conflict between "welfare" and "justice" models of juvenile justice'.

The 1969 Act placed a lot of power in the hands of social workers, and urged the police to make greater use of cautions. Many of the punitive sentences involving custody in borstals and detention centres were to be replaced by intermediate treatment. However, since the Act was so radical, it attracted a good deal of criticism and many of its far-reaching welfare reforms were never put into operation nor fully resourced. Many sentencers in the 1970s believed that care and supervision orders were unsatisfactory and took too much power away from their own role. This, coupled with the demographic rise in the number of young people, resulted in an increase in the number of young offenders being given custodial sentences – the total increasing from around 20,000 in 1972 to approximately 36,000 in 1982. Even so, some aspects of this highly welfare-oriented legislative approach did survive – such as the use of diversionary tactics, chiefly through an increase in police cautions – and became a notable feature of the youth justice system. If the 1969 Act was a legislative high point in the welfare approach, there was soon to follow a clear shift back towards punishment.

The decline of the welfare approach

During the 1970s it became clear that rehabilitative policies were not working. An ironic consequence of the welfare philosophy was that sentences needed to be sufficiently lengthy to allow for rehabilitative programmes to work. This led to a general increase in sentence lengths and to some sentences being indeterminate in length (Davies *et al.* 1995, pp. 245–6). Despite these developments, crime was still increasing and recidivism rates remained very high. What undermined the welfare approach was the realization that custody did not reform offenders and that indeterminate sentencing led to bias against ethnic and other groups (Dunbar and Langdon 1998, p. 13).

The 1970s and 1980s, therefore, saw a re-examination of sentencing policy. In the Juvenile (later Youth) Court, one of the central aspects of the welfare approach was individualized justice, where magistrates selected sentences to meet the needs of the young person even if this meant imposing a 'harsh' sentence. The value of individualized justice was now thrown into doubt, especially as the punishment approach reasserted itself. A renewed emphasis on punishment, summed up as the rise of the justice model, characterized the 1980s and early 1990s.

The development of the justice model

The justice model emphasizes 'just deserts' – that is, receiving a fair punishment in line with the severity of the offence. Thus, in England and Wales, borstal sentences with their element of indeterminacy were replaced in 1982 by a determinate period in youth custody; 'short, sharp, shock' regimes were introduced in 1980–1981 at some detention centres, but abandoned a short while later when they were shown to be ineffective (Home Office 1984). Alongside this was the recognition in the 1980s that custody was not only very expensive, but also ineffective in terms of reducing rates of re-offending. Accordingly, throughout the 1980s, there were further calls for the police to use cautions, even for second and third offences, and there was a greater emphasis on community sentences. Both the numbers appearing in court and being sentenced to custody declined markedly in the period 1982 to 1992 in complete contrast to the period 1972 to 1982. In part this was due to a fall in the number of young people in the general population, and also to the rise in the number of cautions. Moreover, community sentences were seen to have become more demanding and sentencers were accordingly more likely to use them. Finally, the Criminal Justice Act 1982 placed certain restrictions on sentencers passing custodial sentences on young offenders unless the latter fulfilled certain criteria, relating to factors such as an inability or unwillingness to respond to non-custodial measures, the severity of the offence, and the need to protect the public.

The Criminal Justice Act 1991 heralded the creation of the Youth Court and the primacy of just deserts in sentencing. It also provided further encouragement to sentencers to opt for non-custodial measures for non-violent offenders when it toughened still further the community sentences available to the courts and introduced the idea of 'punishment in the community'. Many critics welcomed the declining number of custodial sentences and the liberal use of cautions (although both were soon to change), but the Criminal Justice and Public Order Act 1994 introduced a new form of custody in secure training centres for children between the ages of 12 and 14 in response to concerns about persistent young offenders and their flaunting of repeat cautions (Davies *et al.* 1995, pp. 136–9). Just as the then Conservative Government believed that prison worked in reducing crime (thus ensuring a steep rise in the adult prison population from 1992 onwards), it also appeared to believe that secure training centres would do the same job for children who had hitherto been too young to be sentenced to custody. The Act also increased the maximum length of detention at a young offender institution for 15 to 17-year-olds from 12 months to 2 years. While many of the reforms passed in previous years could be seen as a mixture of welfare and punishment concerns – sometimes tipping the balance slightly one way or the other – locking up such young children appeared to be a most punitive development in youth justice policy.

Cautions and custody: two extremes

The vast majority of children who commit crimes are processed by way of a police caution. In 1994, 86% of known male offenders aged between 10 and 13 were cautioned; the corresponding figure for females was 96%. Of children under 14 years of age cautioned in this way, 89% do not re-offend within 2 years of receiving their caution (Howard League for Penal Reform. Fact Sheet: No. 23). The police caution is, therefore, a quick and cheap way of making many children realize the seriousness of their actions, which also avoids the potentially disruptive and stigmatizing effects of an appearance in the Youth Court. Despite this, there has been great concern about persistent juvenile offenders who, it was alleged, were receiving repeated cautions that had no effect on their offending behaviour. Those aged 15 and above can be detained in custody, and the number of young people sentenced to custody increased by over 27% between 1992 and 1997. The problem, as some have seen it, was what to do with younger children.

The Criminal Justice and Public Order Act 1994 made provision for five secure training centres, each to hold 40 children between the ages of 12 and 14. Those eligible for a secure training order (now a detention and training order) must have committed three or more imprisonable offences and have re-offended during, or broken the terms of, a supervision order. The maximum sentence is 2 years (and the minimum 6 months), with half the sentence spent in custody and the remainder in the community under supervision. The Act was passed by Parliament at a time when there was a sense of moral panic among both public and politicians following the murder of a toddler, James Bulger, by two young children, and well-reported delinquent acts by youngsters on various housing estates. Although statistics did not support the public view of children becoming ever more violent and out of control, secure training centres were presented as the 'answer' to this problematic population. In fact, Hagell and Newburn (1994) found in their research that children who had been arrested three or more times in 1 year represented less than 10% of the population of young offenders, and that only 5% in the sample studied by the two researchers would have met the criteria for a secure training order. Some would argue that the use of secure training centres was a sledge-hammer cracking a very small nut. Critics, such as the Howard League for Penal Reform, stated that the arguments in favour of 'child jails' not only overlooked the excellent work that had been carried out with child offenders in the community, but also failed to recognize that imprisonment was the least successful way to prevent re-offending. Moreover, there were fears that children who attended these centres might learn new criminal skills and that the centres might become no more than very expensive 'schools of crime'.

The debate between the principles of welfare and punishment has been given fresh impetus with the passing of the Crime and Disorder Act 1998, which not only introduced new measures, but also modified a number of existing provisions enacted by the Conservative Government. The significance of this Act is discussed in greater detail towards the end of this chapter and in later chapters.

THE CURRENT WORKING OF THE YOUTH COURT AND THE YOUTH JUSTICE SYSTEM

As discussed earlier, procedures in the Youth Court are somewhat different from those in the adult courts. Usually, the Youth Court is a more informal setting, with the magistrates sitting on the same level as the defendant in a room that lacks the symbols and grandeur of the Crown Court. Defendants are typically referred to by their first names and there is a conscious attempt by the professionals involved in the process not to use overly complex legal language. Specially trained magistrates try cases presented to them by solicitors for the defence and prosecution; they may be advised by a justices' clerk, who is a qualified lawyer, on their sentencing powers and on the proper procedure. Helping the magistrates to reach a sentencing decision – if the young person is found or pleads guilty – will be a probation officer or social worker who supplies pre-sentence reports. With children aged under 16 a parent or guardian must also be in court.

Despite attempts to make proceedings as informal as possible, the Youth Court has been criticized for being dominated by professionals, the so-called 'court regulars', so that many defendants and their families cannot understand what is going on and, therefore, are unable to take part effectively (Fionda 1996, pp. 7–8). Moreover, the Youth Court retains wide powers to order custodial sentences, which diminish what critics say should be a greater focus on community-based responses to youth crime (NACRO 1997a, p. 21). A Home Office study in October 1992 found that 'there had been a slight increase in the use of more severe sentences such as custody …' (Home Office 1996a, p. viii). The report noted that the increase was most apparent in late 1993 when there had been increased public concern about the level and nature of youth crime and impending government legislation, which both signalled a tougher approach towards the problem (Home Office 1996a, p. 51).

Two reports of the Audit Commission (1996 and 1998a) were similarly critical of the youth justice system.The first report noted high levels of inefficiency and ineffectiveness, such as:

- lengthy delays in bringing young offenders to the Youth Court – on average 4 months from arrest to sentence
- too many resources being spent on administration and not enough on working directly with young offenders to confront their illegal behaviour
- relevant agencies working in an unco-ordinated fashion
- too little preventative work being carried out to turn young people away from crime in the first place (Audit Commission 1996, p. 3).

The Commission was concerned by the tendency of the youth justice system to devote its time, energy and resources to processing young offenders, many of whom subsequently had their cases dropped, or who, despite appearing in court, only received a community sentence. This was happening at the expense of focusing on preventative schemes. As James and Raine (1998, p. 94) point out, the Audit Commission's 1996 report proposed a business case – based on efficiency and effectiveness – for redistributing resources within the youth justice system in a way which neatly avoided the welfare versus punishment debate. The report *Misspent Youth* (Audit Commission 1996) and the NACRO report (1997a) *A New Three Rs for Young Offenders*, both emphasized the need to adopt a multi-agency approach to tackling youth crime and subsequently became important influences on the Labour Government's policies when it was elected in 1997.

PUBLIC CONCERN ABOUT YOUTH CRIME

The growing public concern in the 1990s about the problem of youth crime focused not only on its nature and extent, but also on its cost. In 1996 the loss and damage caused by the criminal actions of offenders aged between 10 and 20, and the additional costs of the resources expended by the criminal justice system in response to those actions, were estimated at £5.5 billion (NACRO 1997a). There was also concern that the penalties imposed on many of these young people were proving to be ineffective or counter-productive. For example, 75% of male young offenders released from prison in 1993 were re-convicted for an offence within 2 years, and 46% of those released in that year received a new custodial sentence within 2 years (Home Office 1997b). Moreover, there was a sense that many young offenders were treated too leniently and that a few even appeared to be rewarded for their wrong-doing by being taken on 'adventure' holidays. Of offenders under the age of 21 who commenced a period of probation in 1993, 74% were re-convicted of another offence within 2 years, while the recidivism rates for community service and combination orders were 68% and 76% respectively (Home Office 1997c). There was also unease about the increase in the peak age of known offending, which meant that the criminal careers of young people were being extended. Whereas for many years the peak age for male offending had been fairly constant at 15 years of age, in 1998 it was 18.

The majority of known crimes committed by young people are offences against property, such as theft and burglary. In 1995,

20,500 boys and girls aged between 10 and 13 were found guilty or cautioned for theft and handling offences. In the same year, 11,203 15-year-olds were cautioned for the same offences, and 20,900 youths aged between 18 and 20 were found guilty of theft and handling stolen goods (Howard League for Penal Reform: Fact Sheets 12, 15 and 23). Moreover, it became clear that, based on self-report studies, youthful offending was even more widespread than the official figures suggested. For example, a Home Office study of 1,721 young people aged between 14 and 25 found that one in two males and one in three females admitted to having committed an offence. Although the majority of them committed no more than one or two minor offences, nevertheless, the extent of youthful criminality was wide-ranging, with one in four males and one in eight females admitting to having committed an offence in 1992. In addition, drug use was wide-spread. Finally, the report highlighted that whereas self-reported offending declines substantially for females after they reach their mid-teens, 'self-reported offending for males increases with age up to 18 and remains at the same level into the mid-twenties' (Home Office 1995, p. xi). In 1996 only 11% of all cautions and convictions were for violent offences, of which two-fifths were committed by people aged under 21 and one-quarter by those aged 17 and under (NACRO 1997b). But, despite the fact that most juvenile offending is not serious, the public's impression was of youth crime running out of control. As a result, youth justice policy in the 1990s once again underwent a period of significant change. The main engine of this change was the Crime and Disorder Act 1998, introduced by the Labour Government elected in 1997.

In late 1998 the government then added further plans to reform the youth justice system and to place yet more emphasis on preventing re-offending. Its Youth Justice and Witnesses Bill proposed that some first-time young offenders, who admit their crimes, should have to sign 'contracts' pledging their good behaviour. The contracts may include having to apologize or make reparations to the victim, being required to engage in forms of community work, or taking part in drug-rehabilitation programmes and family counselling schemes. Those who break the contracts, which will be drawn up by youth offending teams, may be subject to harsher punishment including custody.

CONCLUSION

The Labour Government's legislative policies on youth justice owed a great deal to its stance in opposition prior to May 1997 to be 'tough on crime and tough on the causes of crime'. The government was determined to eliminate the confusion associated with the welfare and punishment approaches by substituting a new balance. The new responsibility of the youth justice system was to prevent offending by young people. Accordingly, the Crime and Disorder Act 1998 ordered local authorities to provide youth justice services, and required the police, probation and health services to participate in those services. In particular, the police, probation and health services were required to co-operate with local education and social services to establish inter-agency youth offending teams, part of whose work would be with offenders to address their offending behaviour. Each local authority had to implement an annual youth justice plan, setting out the services, funding, composition and functions of youth offending teams. Moreover, the Act set out a range of statutory time-limits to reduce the delays in dealing with young offender cases, especially for persistent offenders for whom fast-tracking arrangements were introduced (Graham 1998). Finally, and as we have already seen, the Act introduced a new system of reprimands and warnings for young people, as well as creating new reparation, action plan, and detention and training orders.

The Crime and Disorder Act 1998 was the political proof that the Labour Government could be tough on crime and the causes of crime. Courts were even given the power to impose a parenting order, which required a parent of a child subject to a child safety order, anti-social behaviour order, or sex offender order (themselves creations of the Act) to attend counselling or guidance sessions and to comply with any specified requirements in order to help the parent(s) control the child's behaviour. Clearly, the Act was designed to attack disorder and anti-social behaviour, much of which is associated with young people. In addition, the government created a Youth Justice Task Force to advise on multi-agency strategies to tackle offending and on the operation of youth offending teams. The government's intention was to create a number of co-ordinated inter-agency partnerships to help prevent youth crime, and to equip the Youth Court with more effective sentencing powers.

Many will argue that while this emphasis on trying to reduce youth offending is laudable, it is disappointing that secure training centres should have been retained and with them the well-known dangers of incarcerating children (even though as at August 1999 only one such centre was in operation). Many of the government's proposals in the Crime and Disorder Act 1998 only began pilot evaluations from late 1998 onwards, and others were not intended to be implemented in full until 1999. It is, therefore, not possible to draw firm conclusions about the impact of the Act. What is certain, however, is that its provisions will continue to fuel the welfare-punishment debate.

KEY POINTS

- A separate criminal court, the Youth Court, is used to try those between 10 and 17 years of age.
- The court attempts to balance a concern for the welfare of the child with the interests of justice or 'just deserts'.
- A great many children still receive police cautions, now known as reprimands and warnings, and are thereby 'diverted' from appearing in the Youth Court.
- The number of young offenders sentenced to custody has risen recently.
- The reconviction rate for those sentenced to custody is very high and is an indication of the 'failure' of custody to reform their anti-social behaviour.

GUIDE TO FURTHER READING

Both the Howard League for Penal Reform and the National Association for the Care and Resettlement of Offenders (NACRO) provide a number of information leaflets on a very wide range of criminal and youth justice issues. See Useful Websites and Addresses at the end of the book.

Useful information on why young people offend, patterns of offending, and age and gender profiles of offenders can be found in sections of Home Office (1995) *Young People and Crime*, Home Office Research Study 145, London.

In Audit Commission (1998a) *Misspent Youth '98: The Challenge for Youth Justice*, London: Audit Commission, there is a summary of the findings of the 1996 report that sets out what needs to be done, and highlights the government's position and proposals.

There is wide coverage of many relevant issues in Brown, S. (1998) *Understanding Youth Crime: Listening to Youth?*, Milton Keynes: Open University Press.

An excellent all-round introduction to the subject of youth and crime can be found in Muncie, J. (1999) *Youth and Crime: A Critical Introduction*, Sage.

The adult courts

6

Outline
- The adult criminal courts in England and Wales are the Magistrates' and the Crown Courts.
- Both operate according to the principles of due process but are subject to very heavy caseloads and frequent delays.
- Other problems facing the courts include sentencing disparities, plea bargaining, and the differential treatment of black people.

COSTS AND WORKLOADS IN THE ADULT COURTS

The Magistrates' and Crown Courts deal overwhelmingly with adults, aged 18 and above, who are charged with criminal acts. Both courts adhere to the notions of due process in which the rights of the defendant to a fair trial must be protected. Moreover, justice in England and Wales is closely associated with trial by one's peers. In the Magistrates' Court one's 'peers' are the lay magistrates who try the case, and in the Crown Court they are the members of the jury. In this way, ordinary people play a part in the administration of justice and in sentencing decisions, and ensure that these are not wholly dominated by a cadre of professionals. The statistics presented in Table 6.1 provide some insight into the workings and costs of these courts.

THE MAGISTRATES' COURT

With the exception of some very busy courts in large urban areas, the Magistrates' Court usually employs a panel of lay magistrates, or JPs, to dispense justice. These unpaid volunteers normally sit two or three times a month, usually as a group of three people in each courtroom, and are advised by a legally qualified justices' clerk. On 1 January 1997 there were 30,374 active lay magistrates and around 100 stipendiary magistrates who, unlike the former,

Table 6.1 The adult courts of England and Wales – some selected statistics

---

Magistrates' Courts
- cost about £416 million to run (1995/6)
- employed 10,127 people (1995/6)
- tried 1,855,000 defendants (1997)

Crown Courts
- cost about £200 million to run (1993/4)
- employed 2,260 people (1995/6)
- tried 97,000 defendants (1997)

Proportion of defendants convicted of indictable offences (all courts): 66% (1997)

Averages in Magistrates' Courts

from indictable offence to completion:	128 days (1994)
	132 days (1996)
from remand in custody to completion:	53 days (1996)
adjournments per case:	2.5 (1994)
length of adjournment	24 days (1994)
Proportion convicted in Magistrates' Courts:	70%

Crown Courts

prosecuted 89,000 defendants for indictable offences	(1997)
average time between committal at Magistrates' Court and hearing in Crown Court	16 weeks (1997)
proportion of defendants pleading guilty	67%
proportion of 'not guilty' pleas convicted	40%
proportion of all defendants acquitted	18%

Average cost of prosecution (1993/4)

indictable offence	£2,000–£3,000 per case
summary offence	£200–£300 per case

---

are salaried professionals who sit alone in court. Considered to be people of the highest integrity and honesty, JPs are supposed to be drawn from a cross-section of the local community and the group should have a balance in terms of age, gender, political affiliation, social class, and ethnic origins. However, the magistracy has often been criticized for the over-concentration in its ranks of white, middle-aged, middle-class people.

The Magistrates' Court is 'junior' to the Crown Court in that it deals mostly with summary offences, which include most motoring offences, common assault, and taking a vehicle without the owner's consent. These courts respond relatively swiftly and inexpensively (in comparison with Crown Courts) to what are the less serious offences; hence the term 'summary justice'. The court may also handle 'triable either way' offences such as theft, burglary, assault involving actual bodily harm, and some cases of criminal damage. Where the magistrates have tried a case and found someone guilty, but feel that the crime is sufficiently serious to deserve a sentence beyond their powers to impose, they can refer the guilty person to the Crown Court for sentencing. Normally magistrates can impose a maximum sentence of 6 months in prison for a summary offence, but many summary offences are not imprisonable. In 1996, adult males convicted of an indictable offence in the Magistrates' Court received, on average, a prison sentence of 3 months, while in the Crown Court it was 23.5 months. In 1997, in the Crown Court, this had increased to 24.2 months (Home Office 1998d).

With over 600 Magistrates' Court centres in England and Wales they are essentially local agencies. Accordingly, the amount (as well as the kind) of cases coming before a court will vary from area to area. For example, inner-city courts will handle more cases of burglary than rural courts. The duties carried out by the Magistrates' Court are large and include:

- processing around 95% of all prosecuted crime in England and Wales; the vast majority of cases start and end in the Magistrates' Court with only a small percentage going to the Crown Court for trial or sentencing
- deciding the guilt or otherwise of the accused, and passing sentence on those found guilty
- authorizing further detention in police custody for questioning under the Police and Criminal Evidence Act 1984
- allowing or refusing bail
- issuing warrants of arrest to the police and warrants to search premises (Gibson and Cavadino 1995, pp. 24–5).

In cases where there is a not-guilty plea, in order to ensure due process magistrates listen to evidence both for and against the accused person. If the matter is straightforward they will often decide the case then and there without retiring to their private room. However, in more complex cases, or if the JPs need legal advice from their clerk, they will adjourn. On returning to court they will give their decision. Those found guilty may appeal to the Crown Court against the conviction and/or the sentence imposed by the magistrates. Normally it is solicitors, rather than barristers, who provide the legal representation in the Magistrates' Court – sometimes through the work of duty solicitors schemes, which operate to provide legal assistance to those accused who might otherwise be unrepresented.

THE CROWN COURT

In 1997 there were 91 centres in England and Wales where the Crown Court sat, divided into six regional 'circuits'. Crown Courts have more restrictive rights of audience than Magistrates' Courts and, while there have been attempts to introduce more solicitors and the CPS's own in-house lawyers, in the main it is independent barristers who appear for the prosecution and defence in the higher court. The actual layout of the court-room varies from the grand and imposing (not to say, intimidating) to the bland and functional, but all Crown Courts have a number of matters in common.

- Cases are tried before a judge and jury.
- Serious (indictable) cases are heard, such as murder, rape, robbery.
- 'Either way' cases are heard when a defendant has opted for jury trial.
- Serious cases involving those aged under 18 are heard.
- They hear committal cases for sentencing from the Magistrates' Court.
- They hear appeals against conviction and/or sentencing in the Magistrates' Court (Gibson and Cavadino 1995, pp. 30–1).

The Crown Court is the arena in which one can see most clearly the *adversarial* nature of a trial. The prosecuting lawyer (usually a barrister) must present the evidence against the accused in a fair manner and should not wilfully mislead the court or jury. The prosecution must prove the guilt of the accused beyond reasonable doubt. The defence lawyer has a duty to represent the interests of the accused to the best of their abilities so that even those charged with the most awful crimes have a right to expect their defence counsel to act fearlessly on their behalf. The judge must arbitrate between the prosecution and defence to ensure a fair trial and to uphold the principles of due process. Moreover, judges (and magistrates) are independent of the political executive and of Parliament in order to safeguard public confidence in the judicial process. These aspects, coupled with the presumption of innocence, the involvement of juries in the Crown Court and public access to all adult courts, demonstrate the importance attached to a fair trial and also to the maxim that 'justice must not only be done, but be seen to be done'.

The judge oversees proceedings in the Crown Court and handles technical points of law, the admissibility of evidence, and court procedure. If there is insufficient evidence to obtain a conviction, the judge will discontinue the case and dismiss the jury. However, where a trial goes the full distance, the judge will provide a summing up for the jury, but it is for the jury alone to decide guilt or otherwise. When an accused is found guilty by the jury, it is the judge – often with the help of a pre-sentence report – who decides on the sentence. The custodial sentencing powers of the judge in a Crown Court are very strong but community sentences may also be imposed. Defendants may appeal to the Court of Appeal (Criminal Division) against both conviction and sentence. In 1998 there were 97 High Court judges who could also sit in the Crown Court to hear the most serious or complex cases. In addition, in 1997, there were 529 circuit judges (who sit in one of the six circuits), 884 recorders and 360 assistant recorders who were practising barristers or solicitors and who sat part-time in the Crown Court. Circuit judges bear the heaviest workload and conduct the majority of cases in Crown Courts.

The jury is composed of twelve members of the public randomly selected from the electoral register, who decide the case on the basis of the factual evidence put before them. Their deliberations are confidential and, although a unanimous verdict is preferred, the judge may in certain circumstances allow the jury to bring in a majority verdict where at least ten of them agree on the guilt or innocence of the accused. Selecting and empanelling juries is an expensive process and jury deliberations necessarily add to the length of trials. Some critics argue that because juries are unable to grasp the complicated evidence in certain cases (such as those involving complex fraud issues) there should be no juries in such trials. However, the jury system in one form or another is an ancient part of the judicial process and some would argue that it is a safeguard against placing too much power in the hands of the state (Davies *et al.* 1995, p. 188).

Both the Magistrates' and the Crown Courts are society's mechanism for expressing its disapproval of criminality. All citizens, not just victims, have an interest in limiting criminality and in showing their distaste for such behaviour. It is precisely because certain crimes may attract very strong public outrage that we have rules and procedures to ensure a fair criminal justice system. Without due process principles the system would become easy prey to public pressure, prejudice and discrimination. The adult courts strive, therefore, to achieve fairness and consistency. While this is the ideal, it is interesting to consider how the adult courts operate in reality. We go on to look at this next in terms of sentencing trends.

SENTENCING TRENDS AND DISPARITIES

The 1990s have seen a number of changes in the pattern of sentencing in both the Magistrates' and the Crown Courts. The main changes were as follows.

- From the end of 1992 the use of immediate custody by the courts started to rise and has been increasing since then.
- Following the Criminal Justice Act 1991 the use of the suspended prison sentence fell sharply.
- In both courts the average length of custodial sentences has increased.
- Following the 1991 Act the use of community sentences increased, but levelled off 2 years later.
- The use of fines has been in long-term decline since 1992.
- The use of conditional discharges has also been in long-term decline throughout the 1990s.
- The use of compensation orders has decreased in the 1990s in both courts (Home Office 1998b, p. 13).

Despite these trends, which are towards a more generally punitive approach, there remain large disparities in sentencing (Home Office 1998b, p. xiii). Indeed, the Prison Reform Trust (1997, p. 1) referred to sentencing inconsistencies among magistrates as a long-standing 'geographical lottery' despite the various measures that have been introduced to encourage greater consistency. Clearly, such regional variations in sentencing between different Magistrates' Courts is hardly conducive to good justice. The major cause of these variations is the different sentencing cultures that exist in particular local benches of magistrates. Thus, a Prison Reform Trust analysis (1997, pp. 1–2) showed that, allowing for offending profiles, defendants were 'three times more likely to be imprisoned in Sunderland than in Newcastle ... [and that] average sentences vary from 1.8 months in Blackpool to 4.1 months in Swansea'. While the problem of inconsistencies in sentencing in Magistrates' Courts has been known about for several decades, it was only in the 1990s that evidence began to accumulate of the same problem in Crown Courts. This showed that 'the imprisonment rates of Crown Court centres of the same level can differ by a ratio of nearly two to one' (Dunbar and Langdon 1998, p. 69).

In England and Wales there is a tradition of restricting the powers of the judiciary only through the imposition of maximum sentences, which naturally bestows great discretion on sentencers. Moreover, in the absence of much legislative effort to restrict their powers, the judiciary have virtually claimed for themselves the 'right' to have a massive influence over sentencing policy. One way to lessen significantly the disparities in sentencing would be to introduce a comprehensive system of minimum and mandatory sentences for specified offences, thereby relieving the magistracy and judiciary of most of their powers of discretion in sentencing decisions. There might be a further advantage in such a move in so far as it could be designed to reduce the overall prison population. For many years the judiciary has outstripped the capacity of the state to provide prison accommodation, which accounts for the persistence of overcrowding in our jails. Moreover, the judiciary has usually responded keenly to political promptings that it should be tougher on criminals. It was this response, characterized by the 'prison works' philosophy of the Conservative Government during the early and mid-1990s, that led to swift and large increases in the prison population. Thus, in the period 1992 to 1995, although the number of defendants sentenced for indictable offences decreased by 7%, the proportion of them receiving jail sentences increased from 15% to 20% in the Magistrates' Court and from 44% to 56% in the Crown Court as a direct result of the imposition of harsher sentencing. Since no government has felt able to introduce a comprehensive system to restrict the sentencing powers of the judiciary, this country has persevered (somewhat unsatisfactorily) with various forms of sentencing guidelines. Although various improvements have been introduced in the past, the issue of sentencing disparities still exists. However, one could argue that whatever the problems with sentencing decisions, at least they are in a sense fully public unlike plea bargaining which is a relatively closed system of justice.

PLEA BARGAINING

Those who choose to plead guilty (and thereby forego the opportunity of what could be a lengthy trial – and thus spare the system and witnesses much expense and time) will normally receive a discount (reduction) of between one-quarter and one-third of their sentence, although the discount is usually linked to a genuine show of remorse by the defendant. However, it may be difficult to convince a sentencer that one is truly remorseful if one changes one's plea late in the trial, having spent considerable time previously suggesting that witnesses were lying or motivated by malice. Thus, plea bargaining usually takes place following negotiations between the defence and prosecution counsel prior to, or early on during, the trial. In return for pleading guilty, defendants may not only expect a sentence discount, but may also have negotiated that they face lesser charges. Of course, where the defendant is innocent and confident of being acquitted, or where the prosecution has an 'open and shut' case, there is unlikely to be any bargaining since it would needlessly weaken the position of one or other of the combatants. Unlike in America (where it is a much-used device and frequently a topic negotiated openly by the parties to the case), plea bargaining is not yet systematic in this country and such negotiations are likely to be held in private. The pros and cons of plea bargaining can be summarized as shown in Figure 6.1.

Advantages

- The defendant may receive a lesser sentence and/or face lesser changes.
- Court costs are considerably reduced as there is no contested trial.
- Police costs and time are reduced since officers do not have to attend court to give evidence.
- Witnesses and victims are spared what for them is often a traumatic experience, since they, too, will not be called on to give evidence.
- It provides the certainty of a conviction for the prosecution.

Disadvantages

- The sentencing discount, however appropriate in plea-bargained cases, disadvantages those who plead not guilty but who are subsequently convicted.
- Defendants are convicted and sentenced not on the basis of what they actually did, but on the basis of the (negotiated) offence to which they have pleaded guilty, which is contrary to the notion of just deserts.
- The public and especially victims may be unhappy that criminals have been sentenced for lesser crimes than they actually committed.
- There may also be times when undue pressure is placed on the innocent to plead guilty in return for lesser charges and/or a more lenient sentence.

Figure 6.1 Advantages and disadvantages of plea bargaining.

In addition to plea bargaining, another contentious area concerning the operation of the courts has been highlighted in recent times: the issue of discrimination against black people. We now go on to consider this issue in some detail.

RACE AND JUSTICE

Ethnic minorities in professions allied to the criminal justice system

In 1997, 5.5% of the population in England and Wales were from ethnic minorities. While ethnic minorities are over-represented among defendants and in the jail population, they are still proportionately under-represented in criminal justice agencies such as the police and the prison service. Even in areas such as the probation service and the CPS where the proportions of ethnic minority staff are better, they are still not found in many of the more senior positions. Of those with a professional association with the courts, the following Home Office figures indicate the proportions of staff who are drawn from ethnic minorities.

- Just over 8% of both probation officers and other probation staff in post were of ethnic minority origin (as at 31 December 1997). This was actually a very slight fall on the previous figures.

- In the CPS, 8.4% of staff whose ethnic origin was known were from ethnic minorities (as at 1st April 1998), the same as in 1997.
- It was believed that there were five ethnic minority circuit judges, thirteen recorders and thirteen assistant recorders, and six stipendiary magistrates (as at 1 August 1998), a general increase on the year before.
- In April 1998, out of a total of 974 Queen's Counsel – the most senior barristers – seventeen had confirmed that they were of ethnic minority origin; and 8.5% of qualified barristers in independent practice were of ethnic minority origin (as at September 1998), both of which were increases on the year before.
- In July 1998, 8.2% of registered solicitors in England and Wales were from ethnic minorities, as compared with 6% in July 1996 (Home Office 1997d, pp. 31–2; Home Office 1998e, pp. 37–8).
- In 1995 there were no black justices' clerks (Penal Affairs Consortium 1996, p. 6).

Of course, not all probation and CPS staff will work within the courts themselves – nor will all registered solicitors – and some of the ethnic minorities listed as staff members of the CPS will not be professional lawyers, but will fill other less senior posts. Although the probation service shows a proportion of employed ethnic minority staff in excess of the percentage of ethnic minority people in the population as whole, the picture with regard to ethnic minority membership of the senior bar and the judiciary is unsatisfactory. It has been estimated that in 1995 only about 2% of magistrates and about 1.5% of judges who sit in criminal cases were from ethnic minorities (Ashworth 1997). There is still a need not only to recruit more people from ethnic minorities into the criminal justice system, but also to ensure that they rise to the higher echelons of their chosen professions so that our system of justice will become more reflective of our multi-racial society.

Ethnic minority defendants and prisoners

The Criminal Justice Act 1991 required the Home Secretary annually to publish information so that it might become easier to avoid racial or sexual discrimination within the criminal justice system. Each agency collects its own statistics and information with a view to monitoring progress in this area. Added to this information is data from a number of Home Office and other research projects. Taken together such data highlight areas of concern in relation to ethnic minorities and have revealed that although the criminal justice system as a whole is committed in various ways to eradicating racial discrimination, a disproportionate number of ethnic minority citizens are being arrested by the police, processed by the courts, and sentenced to jail. For example, while only 5.5% of the general population come from ethnic minorities, the prison population in England and Wales in 1995 contained 18% of people from ethnic backgrounds (17% of male prisoners were from ethnic minority backgrounds and 24% of female prisoners). Moreover, 12% of the overall prison population (11% of males and 20% of females) were classified as being of Afro-Caribbean origin, which compares with only 1.5% in the general population. Even when the number of foreigners serving sentences for drug importation are subtracted from these figures, the number of black people in jail is still disproportionate (Penal Affairs Consortium 1996). Indeed, in 1996, 10.8% of British males in prison were black as were 13.1% of British women (Home Office 1997d, pp. 34–5).

One response to these figures is to argue that the higher proportion of black people in jail is a simple reflection of a greater propensity towards criminality. But such a view would be mistaken and runs the risk of being criticized as a racist assumption. Indeed, it has been found that both Asians and Afro-Caribbeans are more likely to become the victims of crime than white people (Home Office 1989, p. 47; Holdaway 1996). A large-scale self-report study of 1,721 young people aged between 14 and 25, with an additional sample of 808 people in the same age-range from ethnic minorities, showed that young people from both white and Afro-Caribbean backgrounds had very similar rates of offending, and that Asians had a significantly lower rate (Home Office 1995, p. x). Why is it, then, that there are so many black people in jail?

One cannot assume immediately that the disproportionate numbers of black and Afro-Caribbeans in jail are the result of direct discrimination in sentencing policy by judges and magistrates. Other factors may intervene before that stage has been reached. As we have already seen in earlier chapters, ethnic minority groups are much more likely to be the subjects of stop and search activities by the police, suggesting that the police may be employing racial stereotypes when deciding whom to stop (Willis 1983; Walker *et al.* 1989). Moreover, should the police then arrest someone for an offence, they are more likely to caution young first-time white offenders than their black counterparts. In addition, young blacks are less likely than young white people to admit an offence, thereby ruling out the possibility of receiving a police caution (NACRO 1991). Such an outcome is likely to end in a court appearance, and once in court people of black and Afro-Caribbean origin are more likely than whites to be refused bail and be remanded in custody, which partly accounts for the over-representation of black people in our jails. Finally, a higher proportion of Afro-Caribbean defendants than white defendants end up facing a jury trial because they opt to do so, are charged with an indictable-only offence, or plead not guilty in the Crown Court. Such defendants, who plead not guilty, do not receive any reduction or discount in their prison sentence should they subsequently be found guilty of an imprisonable offence at their trial (Ashworth 1997). These factors also account for some of the over-representation of black people in jail since those convicted in the Crown Court are more likely to go to prison, and for a longer period. Studies on the sentencing of black people have produced mixed conclusions, but we can add more detail to the picture by looking at Hood's (1992) seminal study on the issue of race and sentencing.

Hood looked at information on over 6,000 men and women who had been sentenced at five West Midlands Crown Courts during 1989. In total, the study collected detailed data on 1,441 ethnic minority male offenders, which included 889 blacks (mostly of Afro-Caribbean origin) and 536 Asians. There was also a sample of 1,443 white male offenders. Finally, information was gathered on 433 female offenders, which included 76 black and 14 Asian women. In addition to the factors discussed above (higher proportions of black people appearing in the Crown Court and pleading not guilty) that relate to those individuals receiving longer prison sentences, Hood also found some evidence that indicated a level of discriminatory sentencing against black people, particularly in certain courts. This was not a general and complete form of discrimination against all ethnic minorities (men and women), but was rather a complicated pattern of racial disparities in sentencing (Commission for Racial Equality 1992, p. 34).

Reviewing the available research on race and the criminal justice system, the Penal Affairs Consortium (1996, p. 8) argued that 'there are ethnic differences in outcomes which can only be explained in terms of discrimination'. Wilson and Ashton (1998, p. 89) went even further and stated that:

the disproportionate numbers of ethnic minorities imprisoned stem from profound, consistent and cumulative discrimination at every stage of our criminal justice system, and Afro-Caribbeans are most likely to suffer from that discrimination

However, one of the most recent Home Office research projects – while not designed primarily to look at racial disparities and containing a relatively small number of ethnic minorities in its sample – concluded that:

there was no evidence that black or Asian offenders were more or less likely than whites to receive a custodial sentence when other factors were taken into account

(Home Office 1998b, p. xii)

Clearly, further and more detailed research is required in this area but the strong suspicion prevails that our courts are not free from the taint of racial discrimination.

WOMEN AND THE COURTS

In Hood's study black women were proportionately over-represented in Crown Court cases by as many as six times their numbers in the West Midlands population as a whole. However, they were not subject to higher rates of imprisonment when allowance was made for the seriousness of their offences. Indeed, women, of whatever racial background, were *less* likely to be jailed than men, even in the most serious cases. The study concluded that the over-representation of black women in the prison population was entirely attributable to the facts of their appearances in the Crown Court and to the seriousness of their offences, rather than to any form of general discrimination committed by the courts (Commission for Racial Equality 1992, pp. 29–30). This rather surprising finding, given the numbers of black women in jail, supported the notion that judges act more chivalrously and paternalistically when sentencing women, and place greater weight on mitigating circumstances.

It has been argued that judges and magistrates are reluctant to send women to jail and are more willing to interpret their criminal acts as being linked to medical and psychiatric problems. On the other hand, there is a school of thought that some women may be treated unduly harshly by the courts because deviance in women is considered to be especially shocking and unacceptable. In fact, men and women *are* treated somewhat differently by the courts, but research (Hedderman and Hough 1994; Home Office 1998b) indicates that far from being sentenced more harshly, women are probably treated more favourably – see Figure 6.2.

Hedderman and Hough found that:

- Women commit fewer crimes than men, but self-report studies show that the difference is not as great as official statistics suggest.

- The differences between men and women chiefly occur in the different kinds of offences they commit.

- A higher proportion of women offenders are cautioned for serious offences.

- Current research suggests that women are less likely than men to be remanded in custody.

- Despite differences in the sentences handed down to men and women, women appear to receive more lenient sentences even when previous convictions are taken in to account.

- Women are less likely than men to be imprisoned for indictable offences, with the exception of offences involving drugs.

Figure 6.2 Hedderman and Hough's findings about the treatment of women by the courts (1994, p. 1)

Despite the recent increases in the number and proportion of women convicted of violent and drug-related offences, the majority of female offending is still focused in the areas of theft, handling stolen goods, fraud and forgery (Croall 1998). They are less likely to commit the typical offences of young males, such as burglary and theft of, or from, a motor vehicle (Tarling 1993). The majority of female offenders are cautioned and in 1995 59% of females convicted of indictable offences received a caution, as compared with 37% of male offenders (Home Office 1998b p. 121). Even when women do receive prison sentences, they tend to be shorter than those for men. One of the main reasons for this is that women are less likely than men to be tried in the

Crown Court and therefore they avoid this court's stronger sentencing powers.

VICTIMS, THE COURTS AND JUSTICE

It is the offender rather than the victim who has historically been at the centre of the criminal justice system, and only in recent years has the system moved to satisfy some, if not all, of the needs of victims. The introduction in 1964 of the state-funded Criminal Injuries Compensation Scheme can be seen as the start of a more accommodating policy towards victims. The Criminal Justice Act 1972 gave the courts greater powers to order compensation for the victims of crime. In addition to these financial ways of compensating victims there has also been a growth in both officially sponsored mediation schemes (in which victim and offender are brought together) and in voluntary-run victim support schemes (which help individuals to cope with the physical or psychological effects of having been a target for crime). Victim support schemes developed because many people were extremely dissatisfied both with the lack of information from the police and the courts concerning the progress of their cases and with the poor levels of support. Victims were unsure whether they would be required to testify in court and, when they did end up in court, they complained that they were unprepared for and shocked by what was often hostile cross-examination by defence counsel. In this light, in the mid-1970s, a series of victim support schemes were set up by local volunteers under the umbrella of the National Association of Victim Support Schemes. All these schemes provide support, information and encouragement for victims, especially for those who have been raped or sexually assaulted. Victim Support, as it is now known, has over 370 affiliated schemes and 7,000 volunteers who annually contact about 600,000 victims (Zedner 1997).

Two 'victims' charters' in 1990 and 1996 stated that the police should provide victims with the details of the officer dealing with the case, and that the police should pass on to the CPS information concerning the amount of the loss suffered by the victim so that a compensation order might be made in court if the offender were successfully prosecuted. Moreover, the latest Charter required the police to keep victims informed of the progress of their cases and other matters relating to trial dates, appearances in court, and so on. In addition, the Charter referred to improving provision for victims called as witnesses in court such as reducing waiting times. Research by Plotnikoff and Woolfson (1998) showed that as far as the Magistrates' and Youth Courts were concerned, agreed national standards for witness care had not been met. Too often witnesses were kept waiting for hours before being called into court and the failure to separate witnesses for the defence and the prosecution increased the risk of intimidation for prosecution witnesses. Despite the good intentions of the victims' charter 'progress towards better provision has been slow' (Davies *et al.* 1998, p. 377), while Newburn (1995, pp. 153–4) argued that initiatives that were 'ostensibly about victims of crime were, in reality, introduced because of a paucity of ideas in relation to dealing with offenders'. Indeed, during most of the period when the two victims' charters were published, the government took a punitive line on crime. Emphasizing the harm done to victims was one way to justify a growing policy of imprisonment. After all, if criminals were in jail, victims were 'safe'.

While there has been a relatively long-standing provision for compensation orders for victims, the idea that victims should play a role in sentencing decisions is much more recent and controversial. While it is argued that such a role would give victims greater centrality in the legal process, there is some concern that the inevitable subjectivity of the victim might undermine the objectivity of the court and sentencer. Indeed, Ashworth (1993) commented that giving victims such a role would lead to greater inconsistency in sentencing (and thus undermine notions of justice) because individual victims will have different ideas about the kind and severity of punishment deserved by the criminal.

CONCLUSION

We are fortunate in this country to have at the heart of our criminal justice system the ideas of due process and justice. However, we must recognize that the system does not always live up to those ideals, and that our courts are often subject to unacceptable delays, sentencing disparities and a closed system of plea bargaining. The chief fault in the court system is that sentencers too easily send too many people to jail (especially black people), thereby helping to create prison overcrowding. It is to this penal element of the criminal justice system that we turn in the next chapter.

KEY POINTS

- Adult defendants are tried in either the Magistrates' or the Crown Courts, usually depending on the seriousness of the offence.
- Most cases are handled by Magistrates' Courts, which have limited powers of sentencing.
- JPs or lay magistrates typically officiate in Magistrates' Courts and decide the outcome of the case. Judges ensure fair play in the Crown Court and sentence those found guilty, but it is juries that decide on the guilt or otherwise of defendants.
- Both courts suffer from disparities in sentencing decisions, which makes justice (to some extent) a 'geographical lottery'.
- Plea bargaining and the treatment of ethnic minorities by the courts are both controversial areas.
- Sentencers are becoming generally more punitive, which has led to a large increase in the prison population.

GUIDE TO FURTHER READING

The topics of victims and sentencing issues, prisons and community sentences are well covered in Newburn, T. (1995) *Crime and Criminal Justice Policy*, London: Longman.

For summaries about developments in ethnic monitoring, stop and search activity by the police, the ethnic origins of prisoners, and so on, see Home Office (1997) *Race and the Criminal Justice System. A Home Office Publication under section 95 of the Criminal Justice Act 1991*, London: Criminal Policy Strategy Unit.

There are excellent and detailed chapters on victims, gender and crime, and ethnicity and crime in Croall, H. (1998) *Crime and Society in Britain*, London: Longman.

For further information on sentencing and the courts, and the arguments behind the more punitive approach adopted in the early 1990s see Dunbar, I. and Langdon, A. (1998) *Tough Justice. Sentencing and Penal Policies in the 1990s*, London: Blackstone Press.

Prisons and penal policy

7

Outline
- The Prison Service is very expensive to run.
- Much of its emphasis is on security and control and there have been cutbacks in educational and training opportunities for prisoners.
- Persistent overcrowding, illegal drug-use, bullying and self-harm are commonplace within prisons.
- The role of prisons is constantly under debate: should prisons be used simply to punish individuals and to keep them out of harm's way, or should they also strive to ensure that prisoners learn how to lead useful lives and turn away from committing further crime?

AN OVERVIEW OF THE PENAL SYSTEM

Imprisonment is the harshest penalty available to the courts. However, the number of people in jail is only tenuously linked to the amount of crime and only indirectly to the total number of people appearing before the courts. More specifically, the prison population is a product of the number of defendants sentenced to custody by the courts, the length of their prison sentences, and the mechanisms for releasing prisoners early, rather than having to serve their full sentences. Some statistics relating to conviction rates and the number of people in prison are provided in Table 7.1. We will now go on to examine the Prison Service in terms of how it is organized, the role it serves and its cost.

Organization

The Prison Service, which is responsible for the running of the 135 jails (as at August 1999) in England and Wales, is an executive agency of the Home Office. While most prisons are run by the state, in recent years some have been privately built and operated. Indeed, the Home Secretary, Jack Straw, indicated in May 1998 that all future jails were likely to be privately run.

Table 7.1 Prisons in England and Wales – some selected statistics

Persons in prison:	over 64,000 (January 1999)
Persons convicted at Crown Courts	
Proportion immediately imprisoned for indictable offences in 1992:	44%
Proportion immediately imprisoned for indictable offences in 1997:	60%
Average custodial sentence for persons over 21 in 1992:	21 months
Average custodial sentence for persons over 21 in 1997:	24 months
Persons convicted at Magistrates' Courts	
Proportion immediately imprisoned in 1992:	5%
Proportion immediately imprisoned in 1997:	10%

Prisons are not all the same but are divided into the following categories.

- *High security or 'dispersal' prisons for men* These house the most dangerous and violent prisoners who are usually serving long sentences. In effect, the country's most dangerous criminals are dispersed throughout part of the jail system, rather than being housed in one prison. In July 1997 there were five such prisons – Whitemoor, Long Lartin, Full Sutton, Frankland and Wakefield. Although high security, these prisons are intended to have constructive regimes since many inmates will spend a considerable time there.
- *Local prisons for men and women* These have been described as 'transit camps', in which there is a high turnover of inmates – most of whom are serving short to medium sentences (from a few days to a few months), or who have been remanded in custody awaiting trial or sentence.
- *Training prisons for men and women* These hold convicted prisoners and may be open or closed establishments, catering for those serving medium to lengthy sentences. These prisons may have low-, medium- or high-risk prisoners. Open prisons house those who are not thought to be a risk to the public and include many 'white collar' criminals who have committed fraud, or others coming to the end of a long sentence served elsewhere.

- *Young offender institutions* These may be open or closed and cater for those under the age of 21.
- *Remand centres* These are for prisoners awaiting trial who have been refused bail.

Not only are prisons subject to classification, so, too, are prisoners. The security categories are shown in Figure 7.2.

Table 7.2 The security categories of prisoners

■ *Category A* The prison system tries to make escape impossible for such prisoners since they would be a danger to the public, police or state security if they got out.
■ *Category B* The highest security is not required for these prisoners but escape must still be made very difficult.
■ *Category C* Although such prisoners are thought not likely to try to escape, they cannot yet be trusted in an open prison.
■ *Category D* These prisoners can be reasonably trusted to serve their sentences in an open prison, if a place is available.

Role

Clearly, the major role of the Prison Service is to keep safely in custody those sentenced to jail by the courts. In addition to protecting the public in this way, it also has a duty to treat prisoners with humanity and to help them to adopt law-abiding lives. In addition, the Prison Service must maintain order, control, discipline and a safe environment within jail, while also providing decent conditions for prisoners and satisfying certain basic needs and health-care requirements. It must provide the kind of regime within jail that helps prisoners to address their offending behaviour and prepares them for their eventual release (Barclay 1995, pp. 9–11).

Cost

During 1997–1998 the total operating costs of the Prison Service were £1.75 billion – and it was estimated that spending would increase to £1.81 billion in 1998–1999. Partly in order to contain such increases, the Prison Service had to cut its operating costs by 13.3% in the period 1994 to 1997, with additional cost savings of

5.3% from 1998 to 2001. Between 1980 and 1996, £1.2 billion was spent on constructing 22 new prisons (Flynn 1998). In 1980 there were only 115 prisons in England and Wales, which had increased to 131 prisons in 1996. The total number of places increased by 40% between 1980 and 1996, from 37,900 to 53,128. This massive increase, reflecting governmental determination to portray imprisonment as an 'answer' to crime, has been the product not only of opening new prisons, but also of constructing extra cells in existing jails and of refurbishing old or dis-used establishments. Indeed, at the height of the 'prison works' penal policy of the last Conservative Government, the prison population increased by more than one-third in the period 1993 to 1997. With such large increases in the number of prisoners and despite constant efforts to provide more cells, the Prison Service has continued to suffer from a short-fall of places and, hence, overcrowding. Moreover, the upward trend in custodial sentences handed down by the courts together with the more punitive measures in the Crime (Sentences) Act 1997, means that even more prison accommodation is likely to be required in future (White and Powar 1998). The net operating costs per prisoner per annum for 1996–1997 were as shown in Table 7.3.

Table 7.3 Net operating costs per prisoner per annum for 1996–1997

Category of prison	£(000s)
Local prison/adult remands	20.6
Contracted out (private) prisons	15.9
Dispersal prisons	36.6
Category B prisons	22.3
Category C prisons	17.1
Open prisons (males)	16.9
Closed Young Offender Institutions	18.8
Open Young Offender Institutions	24.1
Local female prisons	28.1
Closed female prisons	24.7
Open female prisons	16.7
Remand centres	19.0

The average cost per place during 1996–1997 was £24,271.

Source: NACRO 1998a, p. 2

THE PRISON REGIME

The degree of 'toughness' of a prisoner's incarceration has varied enormously over time. In the sixteenth and seventeenth centuries prisons were awful places where inmates often died of jail fever, a form of typhus. In the eighteenth century, in addition to conventional prisons, ships (known as prison hulks) were anchored in the Thames and at Portsmouth and Plymouth. On board, conditions were so appalling that they led to efforts by reformers to improve prison life. The nineteenth century saw the development of minimum standards of decency and an attempt to provide prisoners with other kinds of work following the abolition of hard labour. In the twentieth century, open prisons were introduced and it was recognized that prison should make some attempt at reforming, as well as punishing, prisoners. However, even today, conditions in jail are neither satisfactory nor uniform. Local prisons, which tend to have been built in Victorian times, usually have the worst conditions. In addition, overcrowding, generally poor conditions in many jails, and inadequate accommodation frequently mean that prisoners have little to do and can remain locked in their cells for up to 23 hours a day.

A typical day in jail

Today, a prisoner in a closed establishment might typically experience the daily routine shown in Table 7.4.

In February 1998 prisoners spent on average 10.9 hours each weekday unlocked and 9.7 hours a day each weekend. Remand prisoners, many of whom are still awaiting trial (as opposed to sentence) and are therefore still legally innocent, would expect their treatment to be better. However, because they cannot be forced to do work and there is little else to do, they can end up in their cells for 23 out of 24 hours. All prisons operate an incentives and earned privileges scheme, which influences:

- the amount of time a prisoner may spend outside the cell
- the number of visits above the required minimum
- access to their own money in addition to what they may earn in prison wages
- the chance to wear their own clothes and to cook their own food

Table 7.4 A typical daily routine for a prisoner in a closed establishment

Time	Activity
07.55 hrs	Cells unlocked; breakfast served.
08.20 hrs	Those prisoners with work or educational classes leave the wing for exercise.
09.00 hrs	Work and educational classes start. Remaining prisoners are locked in their cells.
11.10 hrs	Prisoners without work or classes are now unlocked and leave the wing for exercise.
12.10 hrs	All prisoners return to the wing and lunch is served.
12.40 hrs	All prisoners are locked in their cells and a roll call is taken.
14.00 hrs	Those going to work or educational classes are unlocked; prisoners with a planned visit are taken to the visitors room. Everyone else stays locked up.
16.00 hrs	Visits end.
17.00 hrs	All prisoners now locked in cells and roll call taken.
17.50 hrs	Prisoners unlocked and tea is served.
18.30 hrs	Access to television, pool tables, table-football and recreation with other prisoners begins. Some may be allowed to go to the gym.
20.00 hrs	All prisoners are now back on the wing.
20.20 hrs	All prisoners locked up for the night; final roll call taken.

Source: Howard League for Penal Reform 1997a

Education, training and recreation versus security

Of course, prisons must try to ensure that their inmates do not escape and, as we have seen, different prisons devote varying degrees of attention to security matters depending on the security classifications of their prisoners. However, it has long been argued that over-attention to the issues of security, control and containment can damage attempts to provide a humane regime and make it more difficult to get prisoners to lead a law-abiding life. Now that the Prison Service has its own business plan, complete with key performance indicators – the most prominent of which relate to escape and discipline issues – it is arguable that the (over) emphasis on security has become institutionalized. Other key performance indicators refer to levels of overcrowding, the duration that prisoners remain unlocked, and to the number of hours of purposeful activity engaged in by prisoners. It is imperative that these latter indicators should not be undermined by an over-concentration on matters to do with security. Many would argue that if security is a matter that the prisons must deliver, there is an equal need to provide effective forms of help and assistance for people who are often disadvantaged in a number of ways. This, it is argued, is not being 'soft' on criminals; rather it is enlightened self-interest, since society stands to gain if prisoners leave jail less – rather than more – likely to re-offend.

According to the Annual Report of HM Chief Inspector of Prisons (1996–1997) it is estimated that 60% of prisoners fall below basic standards of literacy and 70% below basic standards of numeracy. Clearly, therefore, there is a great need for educational opportunities for prisoners. While work, education and vocational training are normally available in training prisons, cuts in expenditure imposed on the Prison Service have meant that educational provision has suffered. Thus, figures for 1998 showed that prisoners spent on average only 4.2 hours per week engaged in educational, vocational or industrial training (falling to 3.9 hours per week in 1998–1999), whereas they spent on average 13.2 hours per week in work and 28.5 hours per week in recreation. Indeed, a 1997 audit of the Prison Service's resources (Prison Service 1997a) found that the level of purposeful activity undertaken by prisoners had fallen in the previous 2 years thereby reducing the chances of prisoners leading a law-abiding life on release.

A 1998 review of the reports prepared on prisons by HM Chief Inspector of Prisons reveals many problems in the provision of adequate education, training and recreation facilities – all of which are necessary to the fulfilment of the Prison Service's goal of ensuring a humane regime and reducing the likelihood of recidivism. For instance, the 1997 report on Exeter jail (NACRO 1998a, pp. 7–8) noted how overcrowded this local prison was, which meant that the majority of prisoners spent little time out of their cells. Moreover, the prison's health-care provision was condemned as antiquated. The 1998 report on Blundeston training prison criticized the jail for its cuts in education, the shortage of offending behaviour courses, the abysmal physical education facilities, and the shortage of work for prisoners to do (NACRO 1998b, p. 4).

THE IMPACT OF IMPRISONMENT

One way to examine the effectiveness of prison security is to look at the number of escapes. Between April 1996 and March 1997 there were no escapes of category 'A' prisoners and a reduction in the escape rate of other prisoners (Prison Service 1997b). In fact, in the 12 months ending April 1998, there were only 23 escapes in total (Straw 1998). But, clearly, there are other measures of prison effectiveness which must be considered, such as the quality of prison regimes, the recidivism rate, the number of suicides inside jails, the treatment of vulnerable individuals and the extent of drug-taking, and so on. These will tell us much about the impact of imprisonment on those incarcerated within our jails.

Self-harm, suicides and bullying

The suicide rate in prison, especially among those aged 30 or younger, is much higher than the suicide rate among the general population. Despite the fact that certain precautions are taken in jails to guard against suicide (such as listening schemes and risk assessments by prison staff) during 1996–1997 60 juveniles held in custody attempted suicide and two of them succeeded. In the same period 65 prisoners took their own lives, of whom just under a quarter were under 21 years of age. In 1997–1998 the number of self-inflicted deaths increased to 74 (which included nine deaths among those aged under 21) and in 1998–1999 the figure increased again to 82. In one young offender institution alone, Feltham, in 1997–1998 there were 234 reported incidents of self-injury and two suicides. Between 1990 and 1997 there were 365 suicides in prisons, including 69 people aged between 15 and 21 years of age. In 1997 three women committed suicide in jail, and between 1988 and 1997 there have been fourteen female self-inflicted deaths. These suicides have affected 70% of all prisons in England and Wales. The Howard League for Penal Reform (1997b, p. 1) argues that 'the isolating and brutal experience of prison is so traumatic for vulnerable people that it leads to self-mutilation and suicide'. The majority of people who kill themselves while in jail tend to do so early in their period of custody, frequently in the first week or first few months of their sentence, which is when they are under the greatest stress. To these figures must be added the thousands of cases of deliberate self-injury, sometimes involving self-mutilation. In 1994–1995 there were 4,778 recorded cases of deliberate self-injury in prisons in

England and Wales (Howard League for Penal Reform 1997c, p. 2).

Clearly, suicide, attempted suicide and self-injury are all highly personal and idiosyncratic events. But one cannot divorce the high rates for all three from the fact that custody is often a frightening and intimidating experience. There are many factors that may push someone towards such a desperate measure as suicide, but the following are likely to figure significantly.

- Prisoners may be located in jails far away from families and friends, who may be unable to afford the cost of reasonably frequent visits to the jail.
- The insufficiency of adequate meaningful activity can adversely affect some prisoners.
- Long periods of being locked in one's cell can have similar consequences.
- Overcrowding, poor quality of food and hygiene, and generally dilapidated accommodation and facilities can add to feelings of depression.
- Bullying or intimidating 'initiation ceremonies', especially at young offender institutions, can lead some prisoners to acts of despair.

The number of suicides stands as sad testimony to the fact that our jails do not always provide a decent and humane regime. We send people to jail *as* a punishment – it is the deprivation of liberty that is the punishment – we should not be sending them there, however unintendedly, *for* punishment. When unnecessary additional misery is heaped upon the deprivation of liberty, we should not be surprised that so many prisoners kill and harm themselves.

The Prison Service introduced an anti-bullying strategy in 1993 and a study conducted shortly afterwards found that victimization was pervasive, with 46% of young offenders and 30% of adults reporting that they had been assaulted, robbed or threatened with violence in the previous month. However, few such incidents were reported to prison staff for fear of retaliation (O'Donnell and Edgar 1996). The study found that one in three young offenders and one in five adults reported actually being assaulted in the previous month, the motives for which included retaliation, settling conflict with force, enhancing one's status, trying to obtain some material gain, and simple boredom. One example of this was in Lincoln jail where in 1997 the Chief

Inspector of Prisons noted the high level of assaults and the endemic bullying in the prison's remand wing where the prisoners had little purposeful activity to keep them occupied on more constructive matters (NACRO 1998a, p. 9).

Drug use

In recent times illegal use of drugs in prisons has become a major problem, which in part reflects the negative aspects of the prison regime. Following the introduction of random mandatory drug-testing programmes in prison in March 1996, it has become clear that illegal drug use is widespread. As part of this programme 57,700 random samples were taken in 1996–1997 and 24% proved positive. In 1997–1998 there was a reduction, with 21% of prisoners tested proving positive for drugs. When prisoners test positively for illegal drugs, they may be subject to loss of remission and, therefore, must spend longer in custody. In 1997 159,000 days were added to prisoners' sentences due to the use of illegal drugs – and this has been estimated to have added £7 million to the running costs of prisons. Whereas drug-testing was found in one study (Edgar and O'Donnell 1998) to have had some deterrent effect on about 50% of the prisoners in the sample, this is not without significant financial costs. Moreover, drug-testing is not without cost in terms of prisoner resentment, for the same study noted that prisoners regarded drug-testing as a means of punishing cannabis use, which many prisoners saw as an overly severe response to what they regarded as a harmless pursuit. Moreover, prisoners generally felt that the introduction of drug-testing had led to increases in tension and increased resentment towards staff.

In addition to testing for illegal drug use, the Prison Service also provides drug treatment programmes on which it spent £5 million in 1996–1997 with an additional £5 million on pilot projects. Included here are therapeutic communities, 3-month treatment programmes, enhanced detoxification units, relapse-prevention units, intensive counselling and education services, and community-linked throughcare programmes.

Prison overcrowding

The fact that some prisons are subject to severe overcrowding further undermines attempts to provide a humane regime, and it intensifies much of the negative impact of custody. Although the practice of 'slopping out' (which involved prisoners having to use chamber pots in their cells overnight) was ended in April 1996 when all prisoners gained access to integral toilet facilities, the problem of overcrowding remains stubbornly unsolved. True, there are no longer any examples of three prisoners sharing a cell designed for one or being held in police cells (as at September 1998), but in 1997–1998 there were, on average, 11,500 prisoners who were held two to a cell designed for one – a 22% increase on the previous year (White 1998). Most of the overcrowding occurs in local prisons, and this adds further to their often poor standards (Home Office 1998c, p. 7).

Clearly, an overcrowded prison makes for an unhappy and tense experience both for inmates and prison staff. There may be insufficient staff to run education and gym classes; there may be a shortage of work; and prisoners' opportunities for recreation may be seriously curtailed, with prisoners, as a result, having to spend much longer in their cells. Such conditions make for resentful inmates and this is bound to make it much harder for the prison staff to maintain good order and discipline, to stamp out bullying, and to get to know and help individual prisoners.

THE COMPOSITION OF THE PRISON POPULATION

The prison population has been rising significantly since 1993. This has sometimes been quite dramatic as in 1997 when there was a 10% increase on the year before, taking the average population from 55,300 to 61,100 – the largest annual percentage increase since 1970 (Home Office 1998c). The vast majority of prisoners are males (just over 95% of the average prison population in 1997), but even this group is not uniform. Among them are to be found disproportionately high numbers of black prisoners, as well as a high incidence of individuals with mental health, alcohol or drug dependency problems. On 30 June 1997 members of ethnic minority groups made up 18% of the male prison population and 25% of female prisoners (White 1998). Prisons also contain remand prisoners, either awaiting trial or sentence. In 1997 the average number of remand prisoners increased by 4% to a total of 12,100, which was almost 20% of the 1997 average prison population. Many of these remand prisoners subsequently received a non-custodial sentence – in 1995, 54% of remand prisoners were treated in this way. Such a number of people on remand clogs up the prisons. An overhaul of the bail system and the greater availability of bail hostels and other supports is necessary in order to reduce these numbers significantly.

The mentally ill

The incidence of psychiatric disorder is high among the prison population, yet prisons are places where good medical treatment is least available and where the stresses of the prison regime may lead to a deterioration in a person's mental condition. Even in the 1980s, it was estimated that about 17% of prisoners might be suffering from a recognizable mental illness. Today, with the enduring problems of community care for the mentally ill (which mean that some people fall through the safety net of community-based care and end up in prison) the position is certainly much worse. In March 1998 the government itself estimated that 20,000 of the then 65,000 total prison population had some kind of mental disorder (Howard League for Penal Reform 1998b, p. 8). Moreover, whatever medical care mentally ill prisoners receive in jail, it is outside the structure of the NHS and, therefore, subject to wide variation in its quality and availability. Only 21 of the 197 doctors employed by the Prison Service in 1998 were psychiatric specialists. Mentally ill prisoners also face long delays before they can be transferred to NHS care outside jail. A report by the Penal Affairs Consortium (1998) found that almost half the prisoners who committed suicide in 1995–1996 had a known previous history of mental illness. It described the locking up of the mentally ill in jail as inhumane because it frequently prevented proper treatment and also worsened their problems.

Many mentally ill people who end up in prison also have a history of having been homeless. Perhaps as a result of their lifestyle, many are imprisoned for public order, vagrancy or criminal damage offences (Grounds 1992, p. 291). This looks very much like the use of prison either as a dumping ground or as a misguided attempt by various authorities to obtain some form of psychiatric evaluation and treatment. However, prison should not normally be employed for such things, and proper treatment ought to be provided in the community.

Young offenders and children

In 1996, prisoners under the age of 21 made up about a sixth of the total prison population – the majority of whom were in the 17 to 20 age range. In 1997 there was an average of 10,810 young offenders in custody, an increase of 12% from 1996 (Home Office

1998c). Between mid-1996 and mid-1997 the sentenced male juvenile population (aged between 15 and 17) rose by 28%, from 1,260 to 1,620 (White 1998). Whereas just over 40% were imprisoned for burglary or theft, less than 25% were incarcerated for violent offences. Over a half of these prisoners were serving sentences of up to 18 months. Of these prisoners, 15% had no previous convictions; that is to say, they were sent to jail for their first offence. More than a third of young offenders had a history of being in local authority care during their childhood. One in three sentenced female young offenders and one in six male young offenders were dependent on, or addicted to, alcohol, gambling or drugs, and over 75% of young offenders only possessed basic educational skills.

Clearly, such people require guidance and appropriate care as well as having to serve out their custodial sentences. Therefore, a constructive regime, free of bullying and containing ample educational and training opportunities as well as counselling and other forms of help, are all vital to any successful rehabilitation. Unfortunately, much still needs to be done, for 75% of male young offenders discharged from prison in 1993 had been reconvicted within 2 years of their release, and 46% of those discharged were given a fresh custodial sentence (Home Office 1997b). Improved rehabilitative work in prison and better after-care and community supervision might well help such individuals. However, one major study showed that sentencing planning and co-operation between agencies to provide help and support was very poor (Howard League for Penal Reform 1998a).

Children aged between 12 and 14 who have committed three imprisonable offences and breached a supervision order, or who have been convicted of an imprisonable offence whilst subject to a supervision order, can now be held in custody in a secure training centre. (Five such centres were originally planned, but only one has currently been built.) In total, 200 places are intended to be made available, built and run by the private sector. The detention and training order lasts from 6 months to 2 years, and half is spent at the secure training centre and the other half under the community supervision of a member of a Youth Offending Team, which are local multi-agency organizations being set up throughout the country. This new form of custody was designed to meet the challenge posed by persistent juvenile offenders who are too young to be sent to a young offender institution. The policy owed much to renewed public fears about the apparently worsening nature of juvenile crime, even though there was little empirical evidence to support it. Whatever the political intentions behind these centres, there are serious concerns that they will prove to be 'schools of crime', in which children learn new criminal skills, which will, in turn, give rise to a very high rate of recidivism. Moreover, in addition to turning policy away from other reasonably effective ways of tackling delinquency (such as reprimands and warnings and community sentences) the new centres are a costly addition to the custody arsenal. It has been estimated that it may cost as much as £2,000 per week to keep a child in such a centre (Howard League for Penal Reform 1997f).

Female prisoners

In the period 1993–1996 the female prison population increased by 66%. Between 1996 and 1997 there was a 19% increase in the number of women in jail. The average female population in 1997 was 2,680, which was 4.4% of the then total prison population compared with 3.4% in 1992 (Home Office 1998c). It may be that sensationalized reporting of the involvement of women, especially teenagers, in violent crime has influenced the courts to become more punitive in their sentencing. About 30% of female prisoners have been convicted of various drug-related offences, but they are also sentenced to custody for relatively minor matters; for instance, in 1995 35% of women in jail were there for fine defaulting. Half have no previous convictions so a large proportion of the female prison population at any one time is experiencing custody for the first occasion. In 1997 13% of female British nationals in jail were black, in contrast to 2% in the general female population. Over 75% of female prisoners have only basic educational skills, and around 20% have spent some time in local authority care, in contrast with a national average of only 2%. Half report that they have been physically or sexually abused, while over 40% report heavy drug use or addiction. Finally, to complete the picture on what is a difficult group to manage, 40% of female prisoners report self-inflicted harm or attempted suicide. Of females discharged from prison in 1993, 40% were reconvicted within 2 years of their release (Home Office 1997b). The position is not made any easier by the fact that while some mothers are permitted to have their babies with them in prison, the majority are separated from their offspring. A national prison survey conducted in 1991 showed that half the women in jail were mothers, but the prison system only contains 68 mother-and-baby places in four prisons for women.

There are sixteen prisons holding women, three of which are open prisons, and conditions are neither radically worse nor better than in male prisons. Indeed, some women are held in separate wings or buildings within the grounds of male prisons, and five establishments currently follow this practice (Flynn 1998). Although much improved now, Holloway Prison was notorious in 1995 for over-zealous security, poor health care, inadequate education and activities, and very dirty conditions. The Prison Service is faced with a fast-rising female prison population, but is not as well geared to meeting their needs as it is those of men (Howard League for Penal Reform 1997d). Women are allowed to wear their own clothes in jail, but security restrictions and financial cutbacks have meant a reduction in the various programmes and activities available for them. Added to these stresses is the often painful experience for many women of being imprisoned a long way from home (because there are so few female prisons throughout the country) with the consequent difficult and expensive visiting arrangements for their families. Young females often fare even worse in prison. There are no young offender institutions designated for girls aged 15 to 17 years old and, therefore, unlike boys, they are held in custody with adult prisoners despite the obvious danger that they will learn new criminal skills from their elders (Howard League for Penal Reform 1997e). An enquiry into the situation of teenage women held in jail found that there was little specialist education, work or training opportunities for women under the age of 18, and that teenagers were expected to behave like adults and were punished when they acted like typical teenagers (Howard League for Penal Reform 1997g, p. 8).

THE RECIDIVISM RATE

The recidivism, or reconviction, rate is the proportion of people reconvicted at least once for a 'standard list' offence within a given period, usually 2 years. Standard list offences include indictable offences but exclude most summary and motoring offences. Some key recidivism rates have already been given, and they are a graphic illustration of the saying that prison is an expensive way of making bad people worse. The latest figures indicate that 47% of adult males, 75% of male young offenders and 40% of females re-offend within 2 years of their release from custody. For males aged between 14 and 16 the reconviction rate is a staggering 89% (Home Office, 1997b). This is failure on a wholly heroic scale!

The factors found to influence the likelihood of re-offending include age, gender, the number of previous court appearances and of previous convictions, the type of offence, and the sentence length. Male prisoners who have served time in prison for burglary or for theft have much higher reconviction rates (74% and 64% respectively) than those sentenced for sexual offences (15%), fraud and forgery (24%), or drug-related offences (29%) (Home Office 1997b, p. 7).

Of course, one of the reasons for the disappointing recidivism figures is that prisons are not very good at rehabilitating people. Once, reformers did believe in the rehabilitative potential of custody, but that idea has been largely abandoned today. Prison staff may do all they can to help inmates but prison requires virtually no personal responsibility from prisoners. Its social and working habits are totally different from those 'outside', and on the 'inside' there is ample opportunity to learn new criminal skills, to become bitter, and for alienation to set in.

It is interesting to reflect on the fact that prior to the introduction of the 'prison works' philosophy in 1993 by the then Home Secretary, Michael Howard, the Conservative Government had actually taken a completely opposite view of the worth of imprisonment.

> For most offenders, imprisonment has to be justified in terms of public protection, denunciation and retribution. Otherwise it can be an expensive way of making bad people worse. The prospects of reforming offenders are usually much better if they stay in the community
>
> (White Paper 1990, para 2.7)

When we look at the reconviction rates, we should remember this statement on the merits of prison, and we should not be so eager to fill our jails beyond overflowing. Despite concerns about the 'prison works' philosophy, it must be acknowledged that it has been a policy with a large impact on the nature of the penal system. Indeed, the apparent continuation by the Labour Government of much of the previous Conservative administration's penal policies owes a good deal to Labour not wishing to appear to be 'soft' on crime. As a society we really do need to debate more sensibly the nature of our penal policy, for on present projections, and assuming that current sentencing trends continue, the prison population is set to go on increasing at what many would suggest is an alarming rate.

The 'prison works' philosophy

Introduced by the Conservative Government in the early 1990s, the 'prison works' philosophy was about much more than jail being an instrument of legitimate retribution. It was about much more than victims crying out for those who had abused them to be punished. It went beyond the idea that prison may serve as a deterrent or have a large incapacitation effect. Instead, it was the very essence of political dogma; in effect, that prison and increasing doses of it were the 'answer' to a crime-laden society. What it did not offer was any rational assessment of the worth of imprisonment, nor any emphasis on the possibility of the rehabilitation of the prisoner. Moreover, the policy was introduced in the face of contrary empirical evidence. There is little evidence that lengthy and more frequent prison sentences are a significant deterrent to crime, since much crime is impulsive and few offenders weigh up their actions with such rational social calculus.

Furthermore, making prison conditions tougher is also unlikely to reduce recidivism, though it may cause further unrest in our jails. The 'short, sharp shock' experiment with young offenders in the early 1980s showed that it deterred very few and that re-offending rates remained very high (Home Office 1984). In any event, why do we persist in talking about how tough jails should be when it is also the duty of the Prison Service to provide decent and humane conditions?

The evidence on the incapacitation effect of imprisonment was gathered by Tarling (1993) who argued that a more punitive sentencing policy would only have a marginal effect on the crime rate, largely because only a small proportion of offenders actually receive a custodial sentence and those that do often receive relatively short periods of imprisonment. Crime is so frequent and varied, and so few offenders are ever caught and sentenced (never mind imprisoned) that custody has a very small impact on the overall crime rate. Tarling estimated that a 1% reduction in the crime rate would require a 25% increase in the prison population – a massively expensive, and arguably counterproductive way to tackle crime.

We now have sufficient detail about the nature of prison regimes and their effects (as well as high recidivism rates) to cast serious doubt on the assertion that 'prison works'. There may be only one way in which prison can be said truly to work, and then only in a very limited fashion – for example, when a burglar is in jail, he clearly cannot be out burgling people's houses. In this sense prison provides a level of public protection through the incapacitation of the criminal in jail. But that is not the sole issue. Just as important is what impact the prison experience has upon prisoners and what happens to them when they come out. Virtually all prisoners do leave jail, since we rarely really lock someone away for life. What is particularly disappointing is that selected aspects of the 'prison works' approach now appear to have been adopted by the Labour Government; namely, its implementation of legislation passed by the previous Conservative administration to impose mandatory 3-year minimum sentences for persistent three-time convicted burglars. We will return to the 'three strikes and you're out' initiative in the final chapter.

CONCLUSION

The Prison Service is under great stress in terms of financial pressures, overcrowding, discipline problems, not to mention the sometimes fragile morale of many of its staff. Current policies look set to continue the massive increases in the prison population that have occurred throughout much of the 1990s. Help is at hand, however, in the form of community penalties but as a society we must also be prepared to use imprisonment more cautiously if we wish to get away from the present situation. This will mean looking more carefully at who goes to jail, and deciding that we should not be locking up so many people who are mentally ill or so many young people; that drug detoxification units may be better in many cases than jail; that prison should be more strictly reserved for the violent and the dangerous; that community-based sentences may be more effective for a whole range of other offenders; and that, finally, it is not in anyone's interests to turn out people from jail who are more criminally inclined and have less social conscience than when they went in.

KEY POINTS

- The prison population does not only depend on the level of crime and the number of defendants appearing in court, but also on the willingness of sentencers to impose custody, and the length of sentence.
- For most of the 1990s the prison population has been increasing significantly.
- There is a high concentration in most jails on security and control, and less on rehabilitation. Recidivism rates are generally high.
- Financial and other problems limit the amount of meaningful and educational activities available to many inmates.
- Prison overcrowding is a persistent problem, as is bullying, drug use, self-harm and suicide.
- Many inmates could be dealt with in a non-custodial setting without putting the public at additional risk.

GUIDE TO FURTHER READING

In addition to publications from the Howard League for Penal Reform and the Prison Reform Trust, there is a host of Home Office material. For further information, see Useful Websites and Addresses.

Issues to do with the prison population, prison disturbances, and the impact of imprisonment are well covered in Chapter 10 of Davies, M., Croall, H. and Tyrer, J. (1998) *Criminal Justice. An Introduction to the Criminal Justice System in England and Wales*, 2nd edition, London: Longman.

For informative chapters on the history and role of prisons, prison policy in the 1980s and 1990s, and a discussion of the 'prison works' argument, see Dunbar, I. and Langdon, A. (1998) *Tough Justice. Sentencing and Penal Policies in the 1990s*, London: Blackstone Press.

In Wilson, D. and Ashton, J. (1998) *What Everyone in Britain should know about Crime and Punishment*, London: Blackstone Press, there are two useful chapters on prisons, including one covering women and jail.

Community sentences: from alternatives to imprisonment to punishment

Outline

- The probation service began in the early twentieth century as an organization committed to advising, assisting and befriending offenders in the hope of rehabilitating them.
- The courts tend to look upon community sentences as soft options.
- Accordingly, community sentences have become more punitive in their content and the probation service itself has had to alter its strong adherence to a rehabilitative goal in favour of a tougher approach.

AN OVERVIEW OF COMMUNITY SENTENCES

Community sentences were first introduced in the early part of the twentieth century with the creation of the probation service. The probation order – the forerunner of the modern community sentence – was rooted, first, in a Christian tradition and, then, in a professional social work philosophy of wanting to help and improve one's fellow man. Over the years, a number of other measures have been added to the range of community sentences, and the professional social work principles behind them have been modified. The social work ideas of rehabilitation originally at the heart of community sentences have now been severely curtailed. For example, the Criminal Justice Act 1991 provided a framework for inspection and set standards of practice to ensure that community sentences became effective punishments in their own right. This 'punishment in the community' approach recast community sentences in a more punitive fashion. It was felt that the public and sentencers would only accept community sentences if they shed their 'soft' image and were seen to become more demanding and 'tougher'. However, whereas in recent years both the Magistrates' and the Crown Courts have noticeably increased the proportions of those sentenced to imprisonment for indictable offences and have made less use of the fine, the use of community sentences has shown only a modest increase. In 1997, 118,000 people started a community sentence under a court order, which was a 2% increase on the 1996 figure of 115,000 (Sheriff 1998).

The main community sentences are as follows:

- probation order
- community service order
- combination order
- curfew order
- supervision order
- attendance centre order.

(We go on to consider each of these in more detail a little later in the chapter.)

A community sentence can only be imposed if the offence is sufficiently serious to warrant it, if the order is suitable for the offender and the restriction on the person's freedom is in keeping with the seriousness of the offence. A pre-sentence report is normally required when assessing whether an offender is suitable for a combination order and a community service order, and is mandatory for a supervision or probation order to which additional requirements are made by the court. Such requirements may include attendance at anger management courses or programmes to address alcohol and drug abuse. It should be noted that community sentences are significantly cheaper than sending someone to jail – for example, the average annual cost of a probation order in 1997 was £2,300. The average annual cost of keeping one person in jail in 1997 was just over £24,000.

The aims of community sentences may be described as follows:

- to deter offenders (as community sentences are now more demanding)
- to protect the public through monitoring and controlling offenders
- to provide an alternative to imprisonment, where appropriate, that is both effective and cheaper
- to rehabilitate offenders through the provision of help, support and additional requirements, which encourages them to confront their offending behaviour.

Community sentences are intended to be disposals for those offenders who have committed offences that are too serious to be handled by way of a fine or discharge, but not so serious as to warrant imprisonment. We will now look in brief at each of the main community sentences.

Probation

Probation orders are essentially attempts to rehabilitate the offender, to protect the public, and to prevent the offender from committing further crime. These orders apply to those aged 16 and over and may last for a specified period from a minimum of 6 months to a maximum of 3 years; they may be combined with another community order (except a community service order) and with a financial penalty. In addition, a probation order may contain further requirements such as stipulations as to where the offender may live, certain activities that the offender must either desist from or actively pursue – for example, attendance at an anger management programme or at a probation centre. Sex offenders, the mentally ill, and those dependent on drugs or alcohol may also be subject to additional requirements (with their consent) as part of the probation order. The probation service has set up a number of voluntary programmes to which offenders can be referred, such as those dealing with drug and alcohol issues and with preparing offenders to find paid jobs.

The traditional role of the probation officer has been to advise, assist and befriend the offender. A designated probation officer plans, co-ordinates and ensures the delivery of the various aspects of the probation programme. However, since the mid-1990s there has been a diminution of the traditional role of assisting and befriending in favour of a tougher regime in which the behaviour of the offender is more strictly supervised and the probation officer is encouraged to report any breaches of the order to the courts. The Criminal Justice Act 1991 brought in a number of changes to sentencing that meant that probation officers now have to supervise an increased number of offenders who are thought to be a high risk in terms of re-offending. In addition, many offenders on probation will be unemployed, have drug, alcohol or mental health problems, or be homeless. A total of 50,700 offenders (the highest ever figure) started probation orders in 1997, which was 3% higher than the 1996 figure. One-third of them had an additional requirement as part of the order (Sheriff 1998).

Community service order

A community service order (CSO) applies to those aged 16 and over, and requires the offender to undertake unpaid work for the benefit of the local community for a specified period, ranging from 40 to 240 hours, to be completed within 1 year. This sentence is only available for those offences that can be punished with imprisonment. The court may hear from a probation officer as to the offender's suitability for a CSO, and the court must be satisfied that work is available. The CSO has several aims, including:

- *Reparation* – the offender makes amends to the community, if not to the actual victim of the crime.
- *Punishment and deterrence* – the offender must carry out work that is physically demanding and involves certain restrictions on his or her free-time or liberty, which is intended both to punish and to deter the offender from committing further crime.
- *Rehabilitation* – the offender performs socially useful work that may have a reforming effect on him or her.

The probation service administers CSOs but offenders themselves may be undertaking a variety of tasks in different schemes which are under the supervision of staff who are employed by other agencies. The vast majority of CSOs are handed down in the Magistrates' Court, mostly to male offenders. The average annual cost of such an order is about £1,700, and in 1997, 47,400 people started a CSO (Sheriff 1998).

Combination order

This order, for imprisonable offences, was introduced by the Criminal Justice Act 1991 for offenders aged 16 and over and is a combination of a probation order and a community service order. It is the most severe of all the community sentences and, once again, is overwhelmingly a sentence for male offenders. The offender may be sentenced to between 1 and 3 years of a probation order combined with between 40 and 100 hours of a community service order. Its use has been on the increase since 1992, and between 1996 and 1997 there was a 10% rise in its numbers from 17,000 to 18,700. Nearly one-quarter (24%) of the orders contained an additional requirement in 1997 (Sheriff 1998).

Curfew order

Again introduced by the Criminal Justice Act 1991 (and subsequently amended several times by other acts), the curfew order may be imposed on its own or with another sentence. A person over 16 years of age may be confined under the order to a specified place for periods of between 2 and 12 hours a day for up to 6 months. The Crime (Sentences) Act 1997 made allowance for a curfew order to be combined with electronic monitoring or 'tagging'. In 1997 a curfew order alone cost on average £1,900, but this rose to £2,700 when combined with another community sentence (Mortimer and May 1998). According to Home Office information, 426 curfew orders were imposed by the courts in 1997. This small number was due, in all probability, to the newness of the disposal, but there are indications that its use may increase substantially in the future as more and more areas in the country introduce the capability for electronic monitoring.

Supervision order

This order applies to children aged between 10 and 17 for a period of up to 3 years and does not require any consent on their part. An element of reparation may also be included in the order. The child is supervised by either a social worker or a member of a youth offending team. The aims of the supervision order are similar to those of the probation order, but, in addition, a supervision order tries to develop the child's commitment to leading a law-abiding and responsible life. This concern for the child's welfare is still a factor in the supervision order, especially with younger children, and it stands in rather stark contrast to the more punitive intentions of the other community orders. A breach of a supervision order may now be punished by the imposition of a curfew order in conjunction with electronic monitoring, which is designed to increase the options available to the court and to strengthen the range of measures to confront young offenders who are failing to address their offending behaviour. In 1997 11,249 supervision orders were handed down by the courts.

Attendance centre order

These orders are intended for those aged between 10 and 20, of which those under 16 can be made to attend a centre for a maximum of 24 hours, and those aged between 16 and 20 for a maximum of 36 hours. Such centres are run by the police, probation or education services and they provide physical training and social skills exercises for the youngsters who must attend. The courts imposed 7,640 attendance centre orders in 1997.

The range of community sentences is, clearly, quite extensive and includes historical elements of rehabilitation (seen most clearly in the supervision order) and more recent punitive elements that have strengthened the operation of disposals such as the probation order.

Finally, the curfew order introduces both an element of punitiveness (restriction on liberty and freedom of movement) and an element of technological innovation (namely, the hope that technology will enable the effective monitoring, and therefore control, of offenders).

THE WORK OF THE PROBATION SERVICE

The probation service, divided into 55 local services throughout England and Wales, is still the most important factor in the provision of community sentences. The traditional role of the service, with its very strong welfare and rehabilitation orientation, began to change in the late 1980s in response to a public perception that the service was too fragmented and that, accordingly, community sentences were not being operated in a uniform manner. In short, there was felt to be too much leniency and insufficient punitiveness in the way these orders were administered. The service is now dealing with record numbers of offenders, as well as providing 227,000 pre-sentence reports in 1997. Simultaneously, it has suffered from a decline in staffing numbers, from a peak of nearly 7,800 probation officers at the end of 1994 to 7,200 at the end of 1997 (Sheriff 1998).

However, the services's work is now to be supplemented by that of other initiatives such as the youth offending teams and action plan orders created by the Crime and Disorder Act 1998. Under an action plan order a convicted youngster may be made to comply with a series of requirements in respect of his or her actions and whereabouts for a period of 3 months. The offender is placed under the supervision of a probation or social worker, or a member of a youth offending team, and will be required to participate in any stipulated activities, to attend certain places at certain times, to make reparations, and so on. The order is intended to be a combination of punishment, rehabilitation and reparation. In August 1998 the Home Office published a White

Paper, *Joining Forces to Protect the Public*, in which it proposed to reduce the number of probation areas from 54 to 42, thus making them coterminous with police force and CPS boundaries. The document also recognized that the philosophy of the probation service had changed from assisting and befriending offenders to one of public protection. Accordingly, the name of the service may be altered to reflect this change. Suggested names have included the 'Public Protection Service' and 'Community Justice Enforcement Agency' (NACRO 1998c, p. 7).

The main criminal justice duties of the probation service are as follows:

- supervision of offenders
- preparation of pre-sentence reports for the courts
- aftercare of prisoners released from jail
- welfare of prisoners still in jail
- provision of accommodation for offenders; specifically, bail hostels and approved probation hostels.

The move towards punishment

In 1988 the probation service was required to draw up details for tougher community sentences and the government also introduced national standards for CSOs, which introduced tougher and more demanding conditions that would be more 'attractive' to sentencers. This trend towards toughness culminated in the Criminal Justice Act 1991, which introduced not only the idea of community sentences being punishments in their own right (and no longer alternatives to custody), but also the notion of just deserts – that the seriousness of the offence should be matched by the severity of the sentence. This proportionality principle was also applied to community sentences, which were now justified primarily on retributive grounds. Probation officers were expected to be more controlling and to have responsibility for aspects of community sentences designed primarily to be punitive rather than rehabilitative. Thus, for example, while rehabilitation remained one of the goals of a probation order, the 1991 Act ensured that this goal became less important than that of punishment. The 1996 White Paper, *Protecting the Public*, argued that above all else a community sentence must ensure that 'offenders have to undergo physically, mentally or emotionally challenging programmes and are required to conform to a structured regime' (Home Office 1996b, para. 7.1).

Moreover, the probation service was expected to work where possible in partnership with non-statutory agencies to provide these tougher programmes.

Further shifts in the traditional concerns of the probation service occurred in relation to pre-sentence reports. The Home Office's *National Standards for the Supervision of Offenders in the Community* issued in 1992 not only stressed the need for stiff and demanding community sentences, it also established new goals for pre-sentence reports. Henceforth, they were to focus much more on the actual offence and the offender's attitude to the offence, with less emphasis on the offender's social and welfare needs. Subsequently, they were also to contain an assessment of the risk that the offender might commit further crimes and of the risk of harm to the public. While such changes were in keeping with the just deserts philosophy of the Criminal Justice Act 1991, at a 'symbolic level, however, they also represented a further repudiation of the social work traditions of the service...' (Brownlee 1998, p. 88).

From the late 1980s these changes extended to the very training of probation officers, with a move away from the existing generic, social work training with a probation 'stream' to a system based on the acquisition of specific skills relevant to criminal justice processes. Mooted in the early 1990s, this system of training was eventually fully implemented in 1998. Brownlee (1998, p. 94) argued that these changes moved the probation service closer to becoming a competence-oriented and managerial culture in which the original humanitarian concerns of the service had been eroded and its application of social work skills were being replaced by a system of offender management. No greater example exists of this than that of electronic monitoring. Even as electronic monitoring was being introduced to this country, the probation service was strongly opposed to the idea of being involved in any monitoring activities. Accordingly, much of the implementation of the first experimental schemes in 1989 and the actual monitoring of the location of tagged offenders was carried out by private security companies. During a second round of trials in the mid-1990s it was found that probation officers were still opposed to such schemes (Brownlee 1998, p. 122), although there were signs that their opposition might be softening. Opposition or no, the Labour Government has said that it plans to extend the use of electronic monitoring on the basis that this form of surveillance will help to increase the protection of the public.

ELECTRONIC MONITORING

Sometimes called 'tagging', electronic monitoring is an American idea that came to prominence as its jail population was increasing dramatically. However, electronic monitoring experienced a number of problems in the USA and, therefore, this country decided first to pilot its use in a number of areas (Worrall 1997, pp. 31–32). In England and Wales the curfew order may be accompanied by an electronic device attached to an offender so that the offender's compliance with the terms of the order may be accurately monitored. Although two sets of trials have been conducted, electronic tagging and curfew orders are comparatively recent and, as yet, are seldom used phenomena. However, it seems likely that curfew orders with electronic monitoring are now being used by magistrates as both an alternative to custody and a penalty at the higher-end of community sentences (Mortimer and May 1998).

It could be argued that any sentence that keeps people out of prison is a worthwhile one. Moreover, tagging also means that specific individuals can be kept indoors (and, therefore, away from certain locations such as pubs, shops and other people's houses) at specified times. The curfew order not only contains an element of restricting the liberty of the offender (punishment), but also it provides some measure of public protection. However, some regard restriction of liberty as an unacceptable imposition on freedom of movement. The physical device itself, which is usually worn around an ankle, is criticized for adding a distinct element of degradation to the penalty (Brownlee 1998, p. 120).

In addition to these moral objections, there are certain practical difficulties associated with electronic monitoring. By the end of 1998, electronic monitoring was still only available in a small number of areas, and there are continuing concerns about the role of employees of private firms in the administration of criminal justice. However, a Home Office study (Mortimer and May 1998) at least confirmed that the technology, with which there had been earlier problems, was working well and proving to be reliable. It is too soon to say whether the courts will impose a large number of curfew orders, and we shall have to wait for the findings of a reconviction study to know how effective electronic tagging is in reducing re-offending – current information simply tells us that four out of every five curfew orders with electronic monitoring were successfully completed (Mortimer and May 1998).

The Crime (Sentences) Act 1997 made curfew orders available to three new groups of offenders – fine defaulters, persistent petty offenders and children aged between 10 and 15 years of age. In 1999, electronic monitoring was extended to allow for early release from prison for some kinds of prisoners under a home detention curfew, with the intention of relieving prison overcrowding. Up to 30,000 prisoners may be released early during 1999 and at any one time this will mean a reduction of 4,000 in the total prison population. Inmates over 18 years of age, serving between 3 months and 4 years, who have been subject to risk assessment procedures and are able to go to a home where an electronic monitoring system can be fitted will be eligible for the home detention curfew. Prisoners who qualify will be allowed out of jail between 2 weeks and 2 months before the end of their sentence; typically, they will have to wear an electronic tag and remain at home (under curfew) between 7 p.m. and 7 a.m. The scheme will be run by three private sector contractors, who may be paid over £20 million per annum for monitoring the prisoners' compliance with the curfew. The government hopes to save about £100 million per year through the introduction of the scheme. Thus, on the one hand (through tagging) the government seeks to reduce the prison population, while on the other hand (through the adoption of 3-year jail sentences for persistent burglars) there will be an inevitable increase in the number of inmates. Cynics might suggest that the former is simply a way of making room for the latter.

DO COMMUNITY PENALTIES WORK?

Thus far very little can be said about the current system of curfew orders and electronic monitoring in terms of recidivism. During the first experiments with electronic monitoring in three Magistrates' Courts in 1989 – which involved granting bail to selected defendants if they agreed to be tagged – only 50 people were made subject to tagging during the trial period. Of these, eleven offended while on bail and a further eighteen broke some other condition of their bail (Penal Affairs Consortium 1995). This was not an auspicious start for this new penalty but it would be unfair to judge it on such limited information. More recent and much fuller data is available for other forms of community sentences.

According to the latest Home Office figures, 57% of offenders given community penalties were reconvicted of a standard list offence within 2 years of the commencement of the order. For probation orders only, also starting in 1993, the recidivism rate was 60%, while the 2-year reconviction rates for CSOs and for combination orders were 52% and 61% respectively (Kershaw 1997, p. 1). The recidivism rates for probation can be further broken down according to the kind of probation regime experienced by the offender. Nearly three-quarters (74%) of offenders attending a probation centre as part of a probation order started in 1993 were reconvicted of another offence within 2 years. For those on probation orders with additional specified activities and those on 'straight' probation the recidivism rates were 61% and 59% respectively. The top rate of recidivism for probation centres reflects the tendency to use this form of probation for more serious offenders with a higher risk of re-offending. Indeed, much of the variation in recidivism rates between the main community penalties can be attributed to differences in the characteristics of offenders, such as their age, number of previous convictions, gender, and age at first conviction. Women and older people have lower rates of re-offending generally than men and younger people, while those with a large number of previous convictions and an early age of first conviction tend to have the highest recidivism rates.

A meaningful comparison of the recidivism rate for community sentences with that of custody can only be made if one takes account of the different characteristics of offenders starting community penalties and those being discharged from jail. When factors such as age, gender and number of previous convictions are taken into account, 'there is currently no significant difference between reconviction rates for custody and all community penalties' (Kershaw 1997, p. 13). This finding is endorsed by White (1998, p. 4).

However, there are some indications that other intensive forms of intervention may alter offenders' attitudes and behaviour and thus reduce re-offending rates. Home Office analysis of programmes run by probation services using cognitive-behavioural approaches suggested that the best results in terms of securing larger reductions in offending were achieved by targeting high-risk offenders and by focusing on offending-related problems. Unfortunately, the probation services them-selves frequently failed to select offenders according to risk and offence seriousness when allocating them to cognitive-skills programmes, and probation officers were also unfamiliar with the methods and theories underpinning cognitive-behavioural approaches (Vennard *et al.* 1997).

Similar cognitive-behavioural techniques were used in motor projects run by the probation service for offenders who had been involved in a number of motoring offences. A Home Office study of 42 such schemes operating between 1989 and 1993 found that, overall, reconviction rates were higher than predicted, especially among young offenders. Only for the older group of offenders who attended such projects was the actual reconviction rate lower than predicted. However, offenders who failed to complete their participation in the projects were subsequently reconvicted at much higher rates than their age and previous criminal convictions would suggest. Nearly 80% of the participants were reconvicted for an offence within 2 years of their original sentence and, ironically, 75% of these were reconvicted for a motoring offence (Sugg 1998). These, at best, mixed results suggest that the schemes had little positive effect on offending behaviour.

Community sentences may be said to 'work' at least in the sense that the probation service, which is responsible for the administration of community sentences, is reasonably well regarded by the magistracy. A Home Office study (May 1997) found that 88% of magistrates were very or fairly satisfied with the work of the probation service in their respective areas, and 90% reported that they enjoyed a very good or fairly good working relationship. Moreover, nearly 70% usually found pre-sentence reports prepared by probation officers to be useful, and 66% were satisfied with the availability of a number of community disposals. As a service provider for the courts, the probation service is clearly reaching high levels of customer satisfaction but, as we have seen, it needs to do much better in relation to its work on reducing rates of re-offending.

CONCLUSION

Community sentences have been busily re-inventing themselves, so to speak, and this has brought about changes in the probation service. The early days of the probation service were about befriending and assisting clients, using a social work model of intervention to 'treat' the individual. Following a period when faith in the rehabilitation model (both in probation and in prisons) declined, the probation service became much more about the control and supervision of the offender in the community. Community sentences also changed and now seem to vie with one another to be more demanding, more restrictive, more punitive – and all in the name of 'just deserts', 'punishment in the community', and 'tough on crime and the causes of crime'. Once, the major role of community sentences was to reduce the prison population, for these penalties were seen as alternatives to imprisonment. Now, they are sentences in their own right. Moreover, probation officers are today more closely tied to the courts, in the sense that as officers of the court their preparation of pre-sentence reports must help the sentencer to assess the risk of re-offending. Currently, community penalties reflect a greater concern for the interests of the public than the needs of the offender. As such, they have moved from being a treatment-oriented alternative to custody to being a more punishment-oriented sanction for crimes of intermediary seriousness with a stress on just deserts and denunciation (Davies *et al.* 1998).

It is not easy to evaluate the worth of community sentences, not least because they appear to have several aims. If the aim of such sentences is to provide alternatives to custody then they have largely failed since the prison population continues to increase. On the whole, in terms of recidivism rates, community sentences do no better nor worse than custody. If the aim is to make available a cheaper form of penalty for offenders then, compared with the cost of custody, community sentences enjoy a great advantage. Finally, when considering the cost-effectiveness of community sentences versus custody, one should not forget that community penalties are in general less degrading and dehumanizing than prison and do not exact such a toll in the numbers of suicides and self-injury cases. In a saner world, we would not be having to justify the punitiveness of community sentences, but the punitiveness of prison.

However one evaluates them, community-based penalties clearly have a future. The questions that may be asked of them are likely to be two-fold. First, can they be refined to such an extent that they actually produce a significant decrease in rates of re-offending? Second, if they are able to achieve the first goal of reducing recidivism, will they ever be able to regain their position as alternatives to custody and thereby help to reduce the prison population?

KEY POINTS

- At the heart of community penalties is the probation service.
- Its role, however, has changed in recent times from one of 'befriending' offenders to one based much more firmly on ensuring the protection of the public.
- The courts, the public and politicians have tended to view community penalties as soft options. Accordingly, greater emphasis has been placed on making them more punitive and demanding as part of the notion of 'punishment in the community'.
- Although community penalties are much cheaper than imprisonment, there is little difference in recidivism rates between the two.
- The curfew order with electronic monitoring is a recent addition to the range of community penalties.

GUIDE TO FURTHER READING

There is excellent coverage of both the probation service and various aspects of community sentences in Brownlee, I. (1998) *Community Punishment. A Critical Introduction*, London: Longman.

For a look at the changing role of the probation service and the principles of community penalties see Worrall, A. (1997) *Punishment in the Community. The Future of Criminal Justice*, London: Longman.

The subject of probation and alternatives to custody is dealt with in Chapter 9 of Wilson, D. and Ashton, J. (1998) *What Everyone in Britain should know about Crime and Punishment*, London: Blackstone Press.

The criminal justice system beyond 2000

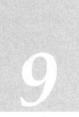

9

Outline
- Two advantages of our system of criminal justice are its emphasis on due process and relative freedom from corruption.
- The disadvantages of the system are increasing costs and burgeoning bureaucracy.
- Even more problematic is the nature of racial discrimination which is endemic throughout the system.
- In this century there will be a greater focus on crime prevention, especially with young offenders.
- Government policies should not be accepted uncritically and the public should weigh carefully the benefits and costs of initiatives in this field.

INTRODUCTION

In this book we have examined the various avenues of the criminal justice system and set out much of the inner workings of its main agencies. We have tried to highlight what the system of justice is seeking to achieve and how it goes about its business by spelling out the objectives of each of the major agencies, and subjecting these to critical examination. Where certain developments have been so recent that there is little or no empirical evidence on which to base an analysis, we have turned to historical precedent to suggest what their consequences might be. In this last chapter we provide a final weighing up of the current system of justice in England and Wales and also attempt to see what might lie ahead for it in the new millennium.

THE BENEFITS AND FLAWS OF THE CURRENT CRIMINAL JUSTICE SYSTEM

The emphasis on due process

No system of justice can aspire to public acceptance unless it is primarily based upon equity, openness, and accountability. One of the major ways to ensure that these factors operate is the use of due process procedures. On the whole, our criminal justice system bases its operations on a clear set of due process principles and, accordingly, receives general public acclaim and confidence. However, no system is perfect and ours sometimes operates in a way that runs counter to the notions of due process, openness, equity, and accountability. As briefly discussed in Chapter 6, the phenomenon of plea bargaining essentially denies the idea of equal treatment since defendants end up being punished not for what they have done but for the 'crime' they have negotiated. Moreover, such bargaining and negotiating are rarely carried out in an open and accountable fashion and run the risk that justice is both being denied and hidden from public scrutiny. In similar fashion, there are developments in the police sphere that also run counter to the notion of an effectively accountable public service, especially in relation to the introduction of new technologies – a matter which we consider later in this chapter.

Relative freedom from corruption

We are also fortunate in this country to enjoy a criminal justice system that is not riddled with corruption. There is no tradition in the twentieth century of judges being bribed to let people off; little evidence of prison governors taking money to turn a blind eye to inmates' nefarious practices; and little tendency among public prosecutors such as the CPS to mount malicious or politically motivated prosecutions. The police still generally operate according to the tenets of public service rather than personal gain and most officers get on with their jobs in a manner that commands public support and respect.

Nonetheless, in terms of corruption it is the operation of the police that gives us least cause for complacency about the criminal justice system in this country. In 1998 over 110 officers in at least seven constabularies were being investigated for alleged involvement in a range of offences, including taking bribes, providing confidential information to criminals and planning robberies. The scale of the illegal drugs industry in this country is now such that huge sums of money can be offered to officers to tempt them into some wrongdoing. Unfortunately, there is a structural element in the police that contributes to corruption; for instance, special investigating officers may be allowed to remain for too long in positions where there are known risks of being subverted by large bribes from drugs dealers, while at the same time also receiving insufficient supervision from higher-ranking officers. In the late 1990s in the Metropolitan Police up to 200 officers were thought to have been engaged in setting up drug deals and robberies. The Metropolitan Police's higher management responded by launching one of the biggest anti-corruption investigations ever. It has to be said, however, that if previous experience of such enquiries is anything to go by, the investigating officers will encounter a great deal of difficulty in bringing such corrupt officers to justice.

We now go on to look at two other flaws: those of cost and discrimination.

Cost and bureaucracy

Clearly, no fair system of justice comes without considerable cost and all administrative systems require a level of bureaucracy if only to ensure that proper procedures are being implemented. However, the criminal justice system in England and Wales has received strong criticism in recent years concerning its growing costs and bureaucracy. Such criticisms frequently focus on the courts (although since the 1990s the costs of the penal system have also attracted critical attention, especially when community-based punishments are so much cheaper). The courts have been singled out not only for the spiralling financial demands of the Legal Aid system – something the government has now decided to curb – but also for the considerable delays involved in the administration of justice. Lengthy delays add not only to the cost of running the courts, but are also a denial of justice. The problems consequent upon these delays are as follows:

- Defendants have to wait too long to be found innocent or to be convicted and to receive their punishment.
- Many people remanded in custody will not subsequently receive prison sentences even when a guilty verdict is eventually reached. Such a state of affairs results in a gross waste of prison resources, creates needless overcrowding in many jails and is an injustice to those who have spent time in custody unnecessarily.
- Witnesses' recollection of events inevitably deteriorates over time, to the benefit of neither defence nor prosecution.
- Victims frequently have the sense that the delays are denying them an opportunity not only to see justice done, but also to begin to put the event behind them and rebuild their lives.

Although burgeoning costs within the court system (sometimes attributed to the fees commanded by lawyers) might indeed be brought under control and reduced, it will not be without 'costs' elsewhere. Typically, these non-financial costs will be paid by defendants, especially the poorest and least educated – who may end up with an inferior quality of legal representation. Governments may wish to reduce the demands on the public purse, but if this should be achieved at the price of lowering the quality of justice, then what purpose is served?

There are a number of ways in which the efficiency of the criminal justice system could be improved. For example, the functioning of the courts could be changed so that they operated for longer periods throughout the day, or even opened on weekends. In addition, greater co-ordination between the various criminal justice agencies could improve operational outcomes and shorten delays. Fewer resources would be needed and less space taken up in our prisons if sentencers made greater use of bail provisions and remanded fewer people in custody. Government proposals to reform the probation service, to reorganize the CPS and to introduce fast-tracking procedures for juvenile offenders may all help to reduce costs and delays. We shall have to wait, however, for empirical evidence before we know whether such schemes are, in fact, beneficial.

Arguably, a more important matter than either that of finance or bureaucracy is that of discrimination within the criminal justice system. Racial discrimination not only denies justice, but also undermines public faith in criminal justice agencies.

Discrimination

There are many people with racist attitudes in all walks of life, but few of them exercise such control over citizens as those within the criminal justice system. This is a particular problem in the police since so much of their discriminatory activities have consequences for other criminal justice agencies, not least the courts and the prisons. For example, since black people are stopped five times more frequently than white people, police activities clearly have an impact on the correspondingly increased proportion of black people appearing in court.

Only 2% of police personnel come from ethnic minority backgrounds (Home Office 1998e), and there have been a variety of studies that have detailed the nature of racial (and sexual) discrimination within the force. Moreover, the police have come under increasing criticism for their attitudes towards ethnic minorities. For example, although the police are now required to collect information on racial incidents, there has been considerable divergence between the number of cases recorded by the police as involving a racial dimension and the number of racial incidents reported by ethnic minorities themselves as part of the 1996 British Crime Survey (Home Office 1998e).

Despite the Association of Chief Police Officers (ACPO) having issued good practice guidance to forces in April 1998 on how they should respond to racial incidents, the suspicion still lingers that the police are not taking such matters as seriously as they should. Indeed, that suspicion has been strengthened and public confidence in the police undermined by the enquiry into the death of Stephen Lawrence. Even as the enquiry was sitting, the Metropolitan Police Commissioner, Sir Paul Condon, admitted that there were racist members within his own force. Although he denied that the police were *institutionally* racist, he nevertheless introduced new training and recruitment schemes to try to counter what racism did exist. In order to make progress in these matters, a Racial and Violent Crime Task Force, headed by one of the Metropolitan Police's most senior officers, was set up in the summer of 1998. In addition, ACPO announced the creation of its own working party looking at policing and race relations.

A report on the enquiry into Stephen Lawrence's death, headed by Sir William Macpherson, was published in February 1999 and took issue with the Commissioner's denial of institutional racism. It concluded that this murder investigation had been marred by professional incompetence, institutional racism and a failure of leadership by senior officers (Macpherson 1999, p. 317). It made 70 recommendations to improve the conduct of the police, chief among which were the following.

- The police service should increase trust and confidence in policing among ethnic minorities by encouraging the reporting of racist incidents; improving racism awareness training; setting out better guidelines covering stop and search operations (and ensuring that all stops are recorded); and increasing the level of ethnic minority recruitment to the police by setting targets for each constabulary.
- The full force of the Race Relations Act should apply to all officers.
- The police should better train victim/witness liaison officers and ensure their proper use in racist incidents.

- Local ethnic minority communities should become involved in the racism awareness training of the police.
- Racist language or conduct by an officer should normally merit dismissal from the police (Macpherson 1999, pp. 327–35).

The Metropolitan Police's decision to set up their racial task force and to review recruitment practices and was not simply a tactic to dilute impending criticism from the Macpherson enquiry, but was an attempt to alter the culture of the police, which the head of the Police Complaints Authority has referred to as a culture of racism (*The Independent*, 15 August 1998, p. 11). Whether the efforts made by the Metropolitan Police and ACPO, the recommendations of the Macpherson report, and a Home Office decision to insist that all constabularies recruit more ethnic minority officers will bring about significant change remains to be seen. Strong action has to be taken to turn our police into agencies free of racism and to restore public confidence, especially among ethnic minorities themselves. The police might, for example, discriminate less if racists could be detected at the recruitment stage. None of this is intended to suggest that all officers, or even the majority, are racists. Furthermore, much racist conduct may be unintentional and it is to be hoped that improved training will eradicate it. What *is* clear is that any racist action on the part of the police, even if carried out by relatively few officers, has widespread and deleterious consequences for the quality of justice and for the standing of the police.

Increasing costs, bureaucratic delays and discrimination are all clearly visible within the criminal justice system, and their deleterious consequences are all too easily recognizable. So, what are some of the major options that the criminal justice system in this century could pursue?

OPTIONS FOR THE NEW MILLENNIUM

A Ministry of Justice

At present, political and administrative responsibility for criminal justice agencies in England and Wales is split – so that just as there are difficulties in ensuring operational co-ordination between these agencies, there is also a problem about overall policy planning and implementation. Frequently, what happens in one agency has consequences for other agencies. For instance, the CPS's guidelines on what is acceptable evidence and what prosecutions may or may not be in the public interest have clear implications for the police and the way in which they act. For many years, police complaints about the operation of the CPS and the high number of discontinued cases fell on deaf political ears. Even if these complaints had been taken up by the police's political 'masters', the Home Office, the matter could not have been dealt with internally since the Home Office would have had to speak to the separate government department that has responsibility for the CPS. Likewise, when the courts sentence significantly more people to custody – even though they may be following government policy such as the 'prison works' philosophy – they create immense difficulties for the penal system. Again, two government departments are involved here and, although they may serve the same political party in power, government departments do not always have similar or even over-lapping interests. Resolving conflicts of interest can be difficult and time-consuming, especially when their resolution may depend on receiving extra resources (which are extremely scarce and often the subject of bitter inter-departmental competition).

As a result of this situation, there is now some argument in favour of pursuing a co-ordinated set of criminal justice policies through the creation of a Ministry of Justice with responsibility for all criminal justice agencies. This would allow for the consequences of certain policies for criminal justice agencies to be discussed – and then, if necesary, for those policies to be altered at an early planning stage. Moreover, the monitoring of policy implementation could be expedited and appropriate remedial action taken more quickly. This would not mean surrendering the operational independence of the police and the judiciary, but it might mean that criminal justice policy in this country would be better conceived and implemented. A concept of a Ministry of Justice deserves serious consideration, but there are other matters (less radical in political terms than the creation of such a ministry) that must also be addressed.

Greater focus on crime prevention

Crime prevention has often been the poor relation of 'sexier' operations such as crime detection using specialist squads and high-tech equipment, or else has lagged in public appeal behind the 'hang 'em and flog 'em' brigade, whose direct approach to solving crime appeals to those desperate for any kind of solution. Crime prevention does, however, deserve much greater attention.

There are at least four broad types of crime prevention, examples of which may sometimes overlap these categories. These categories are:

- *Traditional crime prevention* which incorporates an emphasis on disseminating knowledge and information designed to make it harder to steal things. This target-hardening approach includes the police and local authorities in giving advice on fitting more effective locks and special initiatives by the police to encourage people to mark their property with 'invisible' identification information.
- *Operational crime prevention* which is practised through schemes such as neighbourhood watch and efforts by the police and other agencies to provide practical help to repeat victims. Some community policing schemes and intelligence-led operations might also be included here.
- *Technological crime prevention* which, with its reliance on electronic and technological developments to deter crime, makes it harder to commit crime and easier to detect it. Included here would be the various developments in car security, better lighting in public places and, perhaps most importantly, CCTV (closed-circuit television).
- *Social crime prevention* which goes far beyond the responsibilities of the police and embraces policies that we might not normally associate with preventing crime – such as the provision of some additional form of schooling or job training for those in need. It might also embrace better employment and housing opportunities.

At present, crime prevention in this country is an amalgam of all four of the above categories. However, it is the *social* element of crime prevention that has typically been overlooked. Sometimes such policies are seen as either too radical or else too expensive; and sometimes they are viewed somehow as denying 'just deserts' to criminals. 'Why should we do more for criminals and potential criminals than we do for the law-abiding?' runs the argument. It is a false argument, and divisive, for it assumes we must place a greater value on some citizens than on others. The point here is not differential worth but the rights of *all* citizens to decent minimum standards in modern-day necessities – education, accommodation, employment, and so on. As an example of the value of this social approach to crime prevention, we now consider the problem of young people and crime.

YOUNG PEOPLE AND CRIME PREVENTION

Youth crime in this country is serious. It is estimated that 7 million offences are committed annually by young people, only 19% of which are officially recorded by the police. Moreover, people under the age of 21 are responsible for about half of all recorded crime, which is estimated to cost society around £13 billion. Young criminals can also be among the most prolific, with around 17% of persistent offenders being responsible for 60% of all crime. Just as alarmingly, young men are extending their criminal careers into their twenties and are not abandoning crime after their teenage years as was the case for most offenders previously. Ironically, young people are also the most frequent *victims* of crime (Bright 1998, p. 15).

There is no single cause of youth crime and, therefore, there can be no single solution. What is required is a wide-ranging approach adopting a variety of measures. Bright (1998) suggested that the following eight measures should be promoted and, indeed, the present government is now actively pursuing many of them. These measures are:

- improve the quality of parenting through parenting programmes, leading to better behaviour on the part of the child
- prevent failure at school since unsuccessful or disruptive pupils are more likely to truant and become involved in crime (in particular, better pre-school education and family literacy projects will be required; American research suggests that for every $1 invested in these kinds of educational projects, some $7 are saved in future criminal costs)
- target youth work in priority areas and focus on those youngsters most in need
- prepare youngsters for employment through training schemes and other supportive projects
- tackle drug abuse and, thus, cut down the number of drug-related crimes
- reduce nuisance and disorder among young people through youth work projects, problem-oriented policing and neighbourhood mediation services
- make it harder to commit crime by improving the design, security and policing of those places where young people tend to gather and, hence, reduce the levels of repeat victimization
- prevent repeat offending by targeting likely offenders and providing them with intensive and rigorous community sentences.

Not only is such an approach more innovative than relying on a punitive response to youth crime, but it is also a *long-term* strategy. If it is to be successful then it must be implemented and refined over a number of years. It appears as if the Labour Government is prepared to adopt such a strategy.

CONCLUSION

In 1998 the government launched a £250 million initiative to develop an effective crime reduction strategy, including £50 million to be used to provide alarms for the 2 million homes in Britain facing the highest risks of burglary. As further proof of its determination to tackle crime, in 1999 the Home Office announced a £60 million crime reduction scheme, much of which will depend on encouraging companies to design their products with crime prevention in mind – for example, installing security chips in electronic goods. The government's initiatives range across all four kinds of crime prevention and are an integral part of its promise 'to be tough on crime and the causes of crime'. One example of this promise was contained in the Crime and Disorder Act 1998, which places a duty on the police and local authorities to draw up local community safety plans. The Act will also lead to an overhaul of the youth justice system with a focus on reducing offending. In keeping with some of the eight measures outlined by Bright (1998) that we have just looked at, the Crime and Disorder Act contains a number of relevant provisions. These include:

- reparation and action plan orders for young people to try to turn them away from crime
- youth offending teams and youth justice plans to tackle delinquency in local areas
- anti-social behaviour orders for anyone aged 10 or over to reduce harassment and actions that cause harm and distress
- parenting orders to improve parenting skills
- local child curfew schemes, which may ban unsupervised children aged under 10 from being outside their homes between certain times.

The attempt to control crime has enjoyed three phases in recent times. In the 1970s the prevailing view was that 'nothing works' in terms of significantly reducing crime and so the country struggled along with rather traditional approaches to criminality.

The next major shift in the early 1990s was the over-simplistic assertion that 'prison works'. This policy of locking up more and more people was enthusiastically followed during much of the last Conservative Government's period in office. Many professionals involved in criminal justice hoped for a more enlightened approach from the Labour Government elected in May 1997. The Crime and Disorder Act 1998, one of Labour's flagship policies in this field, received a mixed welcome. Critics of the Act have pointed to a touch of authoritarianism in its approach. Others point to its robust common sense. Whatever one's view, it is clear that this Act contains a heavy emphasis on crime reduction and prevention and has ushered in a third phase in the battle against crime. Although some will be unhappy at the introduction of mandatory minimum 3-year sentences for repeat burglars and the retention of secure training centres, this new approach does, at least, seem to be a set of inter-related policies that attempt to tackle crime on a wide front. Moreover, for the first time, much government policy is firmly based on research findings – something that had, hitherto, largely been ignored!

There are a number of current policies that look as if they will be increasingly favoured by the government, and about which some care will need to be exercised. Among them is zero tolerance. Although this approach was hailed as a great success when introduced in New York, only a few years later in 1999 there were growing suspicions that some patrol officers were acting too aggressively and harassing black people in the name of this kind of policing. Herein lies a danger. Many initiatives to tackle crime are glibly labelled by the media or else touted by politicians as a quick fix to a problem. We do the public no favours when all we put before them are slogans such as 'zero tolerance' with its implied promise of salvation. Zero tolerance policing will not 'solve' crime and we should not allow it to become widespread simply on the assumption that it will. Empirical enquiry will tell us how well or otherwise zero tolerance policing reduces crime in this country but in the meantime we must guard against this form of policing being used as just another stick with which to beat groups whom the police dislike or wish to discipline. Down that road lies disorder and resentment, not salvation.

The increased use of technology is another idea frequently put forward as a solution to the problem of crime. Many people accept without demur the proliferation of cameras in public and private places because we are told that CCTV will deter criminals. Perhaps it may do so, but what is less well known is the underside of technology. One report (NACRO 1997b) found that many CCTV cameras were being used selectively and disproportionately to target young, black males – not because of any alleged involvement in wrong-doing, but simply because of the camera operator's own prejudices about whom to focus on. Similar unintended consequences of the introduction of new technology have arisen following the issuing of CS gas sprays to most patrol officers in England and Wales. Although these sprays were given to officers to help protect themselves against violent attack, the Police Complaints Authority has now warned that some unfit, middle-aged officers are using the sprays wrongly in order to make an arrest and to avoid having to use other restraint methods (*The Independent*, 12 August 1998, p. 4). There are suspicions that the spray has replaced the truncheon as the first line of defence even though the gas is supposed to be used only in extreme circumstances when an officer is under direct physical threat.

Both CCTV and the use of CS gas are examples of areas in which constant public vigilance is needed to ensure that public bodies, even if acting in the public's name, do not abuse their powers. The public should be given better and more detailed information about these policies so that they can judge whether or not such tactics are worth pursuing; this means knowing about costs as well as the benefits. Governments must play their part in making this information available. Furthermore, although they cannot completely ignore the views of the public, the government should avoid constantly pandering to populist notions. For example, the governmental desire to change the name of the probation service to something along the lines of the Public Protection Service strongly suggests an attempt at 're-branding' rather than effective re-organization. Where does this end? Are we so desperate to appease the public on matters to do with crime that prisons will soon be re-branded 'torture chambers'?

It is essential that toughness is not confused with effectiveness. There will always be some criminals for whom punishment and imprisonment is the appropriate option. However, this does not mean that criminal justice agencies need to be tougher on *all* offenders. What these agencies need to be is more effective, and achieving that goal requires thoughtful planning and careful consideration – not slogans and quick fixes.

KEY POINTS

- Our criminal justice system emphasizes due process and is relatively free of corruption.
- The system is, however, overly bureaucratic and costly to run.
- Racial discrimination within the system, especially within the police, undermines justice and the public's confidence in the agencies of law and order.
- Administrative responsibility for the agencies is fragmented and the idea of a Ministry of Justice is therefore worthy of consideration.
- Government policies now increasingly focus on crime prevention.
- All policies have costs and unintended consequences as well as benefits; the public need to weigh up the pros and cons critically.

GUIDE TO FURTHER READING

The following references contain material on the future direction of the criminal justice system and its agencies, or else provide a critique of existing arrangements.

Stephens, M. and Becker, S. (1994) *Police Force, Police Service. Care and Control in Britain*. London: Macmillan.

Wilson, D. and Ashton, J. (1998) *What Everyone in Britain should know about Crime and Punishment*, London: Blackstone Press.

Leishman, F., Loveday, B. and Savage, S. (1996) *Core Issues in Policing*, London: Longman.

Davies, M., Croall, H. and Tyrer, J. (1998) *Criminal Justice. An Introduction to the Criminal Justice System in England and Wales*. London: Longman, 2nd edition.

Crawford, A. (1998) *Crime Prevention and Community Safety: Politics, Policies and Practices*, Harlow: Longman.

Matthews, R. and Francis, P. (eds) (1996) *Prisons 2000: An International Perspective on the Current State and Future of Imprisonment*, Basingstoke: Macmillan.

Appendix

It is very important that students of crime and social policy are familiar with the most recent official statistical data. In a book of this size, it is not possible to include large amounts of such data, which is in any case readily available in the following publications:

- *Social Trends*
- *Key Data*
- *Criminal Statistics.*

These three are all published annually by The Stationery Office (0870 6005522). They will be available in most reference libraries.

- *The British Crime Survey.*

This is published by the Home Office. The most recent version is dated 1998. Selected tables appear in *Social Trends* and in *Key Data*.
The Office for National Statistics is building a website at *http://www.ons.gov.uk/index.htm.* You may find the 'United Kingdom in Figures' and 'Statbase' sections useful. At the time of writing the 'Bookshelf' section included an inactive link to Crime and Justice, but it may be worth checking from time to time in case it is activated.

The tables that appear below are included in this book to provide a broad background and are only a starting-point for further study.

Table 1.1 Notifiable offences recorded by the police: by type of offence

	England and Wales			Scotland			Northern Ireland		
	1981	1991	1997	1981	1991	1997	1981	1991	1997[1]
Theft and handling stolen goods,	1,603	2,761	2,165	201	284	188	25	32	30
of which: theft of vehicles	333	582	407	33	44	29	5	8	9
theft from vehicles	380	913	710	–	–	52	7	7	5
Burglary	718	1,219	1,015	96	116	55	20	17	14
Criminal damage[2]	387	821	877	62	90	81	5	2	5
Violence against the person	100	190	251	8	16	15	3	4	5
Fraud and forgery	107	175	134	21	26	21	3	5	4
Robbery	20	45	63	4	6	4	3	2	2
Sexual offences,	19	29	33	2	3	4	–	1	1
of which: rape	1	4	7	–	1	1	–	–	–
Drug trafficking	–	11	23	2	3	8	–	–	–
Other notifiable offences[3]	9	23	37	12	28	43	3	1	1
All notifiable offences	2,964	5,276	4,598	408	573	421	62	64	62

1 No longer includes assault on police and communicating false information regarding a bomb hoax. These offences have been removed from the categories 'Violence against the person' and 'Other notifiable offences'.

2 In Northern Ireland excludes criminal damage valued at less than £200.

3 In Northern Ireland includes 'possession of controlled drugs' and 'offences against the state'. In Scotland excludes 'offending while on bail' from 1991 onwards.

Source: Home Office; The Scottish Office Home Department; Royal Ulster Constabulary

Table 1.2 Offenders found guilty of, or cautioned for, indictable offences: by gender, type of offence and age, 1997

England and Wales	Rates per 10,000 population				
	10–15	16–24	25–34	35 and over	All aged 10 and over (thousands)
Males					
Theft and handling stolen goods	124	216	85	18	149
Drug offences	12	158	63	8	86
Violence against the person	30	71	32	7	50
Burglary	43	71	18	2	39
Criminal damage	11	18	7	1	12
Robbery	6	11	2	–	6
Sexual offences	3	4	3	2	6
Other indictable offences	11	101	59	11	72
All indictable offences	240	651	269	50	420
Females					
Theft and handling stolen goods	58	70	30	7	52
Drug offences	1	17	9	1	10
Violence against the person	11	11	5	1	9
Burglary	3	3	1	–	2
Criminal damage	1	2	1	–	1
Robbery	1	1	–	–	1
Sexual offences	–	–	–	–	–
Other indictable offences	3	18	12	2	13
All indictable offences	80	122	57	11	88

Source: Home Office

Table 1.3 Number of crimes estimated by the BCS in 1997

	Number of crimes in thousands
Vandalism (against vehicles and other private property)	**2,917**
All property thefts	**10,134**
Burglary (actual and attempted)	1,639
Vehicle related thefts (thefts of, from and attempts)	3,483
Bicycle thefts	549
Other household thefts	2,067
Other personal thefts (including stealth thefts)	2,397
All violence	**3,381**
Mugging (robbery and snatch thefts)	390
Wounding	714
Common assault	2,276
All BCS crime	**16,437**

Source: The British Crime Survey England and Wales, Home Office 1998

Note: Subtotals do not add to total due to rounding.

Table 1.4 Proportion of adult victims of violence by household characteristics 1998

	% victims once or more				
	All violence	Domestic	Acquaintance	Stranger	Mugging
Head of household under 60					
Single adult and child(ren)	11.9	6.9	3.0	1.4	0.9
Adults and child(ren)	5.6	1.0	2.4	1.5	1.0
No children	6.0	0.8	3.0	1.8	1.0
Head of household over 60	1.2	0.1	0.5	0.3	0.4
Household income (£)					
<5k	6.6	1.9	2.5	1.4	1.5
5k<10k	2.9	0.9	1.1	0.6	0.6
10k<20k	4.1	0.9	2.0	1.0	0.6
20k<30k	4.7	0.4	1.9	1.9	0.9
30k+	5.1	0.6	2.6	1.3	0.8
Tenure					
Owner occupiers	3.2	0.4	1.4	1.0	0.5
Social renters	6.3	1.8	2.6	1.4	1.2
Private renters	9.4	2.1	4.2	2.5	1.4
Accommodation type					
Houses	4.5	0.9	2.0	1.3	0.6
Detached	3.1	0.5	1.4	0.7	0.8
Semi-detached	4.1	0.9	1.8	1.2	0.4
Mid terrace	5.9	1.1	2.7	1.8	0.7
End terrace	6.3	1.4	2.3	2.2	1.5
Flats/maisonettes	6.4	0.9	2.8	1.3	1.9
All adults	**4.7**	**0.9**	**2.1**	**1.3**	**0.8**

Source: The 1998 British Crime Survey England and Wales, Home Office 1998

Useful websites
and addresses

WEBSITES

Judiciary and the courts

Website: *http://www.open.gov.uk/lcd/*
Here you can find information on legal aid, the courts, lawyers, judges (including recent appointments), magistrates (including their duties and responsibilities), the Crown Prosecution Service, and other related criminal matters.

Crown Prosecution Service

Website: *http://www.cps.gov.uk*
The site contains information on the role and work of the CPS and where it is located. It also outlines its policies towards the treatment of victims and witnesses, and towards the prosecution of cases of domestic violence. There are instructions on how to obtain a VHS-format video of the work of the service, and on how to download a series of video clips. (This site may also be accessed from the Lord Chancellor's Department's site which is listed under 'The Judiciary and the Courts' above.

The prisons

Website: *http://www.open.gov.uk/prison/prisonhm.htm*
This site is exclusively about the uses of psychology in prisons, including a section on the bullying of young offenders. If you want a career as a psychologist working in a prison, this is the website for you!

The Metropolitan Police

Website: *http://www.met.police.uk/*
This is an excellent site with a lot of information on a large number of topics, including the annual report, Operations Bumblebee and Eagle Eye to combat burglaries and street robberies, neighbourhood watch, and a description of what the police do and how they are organized. You can also access many other UK police forces by clicking on the 'POLICE UK' logo on the Quick Index page.

Statistical data

Website: *http://www.homeoffice.gov.uk/rds/index.htm*
Here you can find information and statistical data on a large number of topics, including recorded crime, the British Crime Survey, probation, drug offences, prison population, and so on.

The Home Office

Website: *http://www.homeoffice.gov.uk/*
This is another very useful site from which you can obtain information on recent developments in the criminal justice area, crime and drug prevention, the Crime and Disorder Act 1998, and material about the latest publications. There is also a very good search facility, which allows you to download and read many of the Home Office publications thrown up by the search engine as being relevant to your query.

Crime Prevention
The following websites contain information on crime prevention, from national and international sources.
Website: *http://www.homeoffice.gov.uk/cpa.htm*
http://www.crime-prevention-intl.org/
http://www.ncjrs.org/cpwww.htm

ADDRESSES

The Home Office

A large number of research studies and statistical bulletins may be obtained free of charge from:
Research, Development and
Statistics Directorate
Information and Publications
Group
Room 201, Home Office
50 Queen Anne's Gate
London SW1H 9AT

NACRO

For information on the courts, probation, prisons and the criminal justice system in general, contact:
NACRO
169 Clapham Rd
London SW9 0PU
Tel: 0171 582 6500

The Metropolitan Police

Enquiries may be addressed to:
Metropolitan Police
Directorate of Public Affairs
Scotland Yard
10, Broadway
London SW1H OBG
Tel: 0171 230 1212

The Audit Commission

This organization produces a number of occasional reports on police activities and annual reports on police performance indicators. Contact:
AuditCommission Publications
Bookpoint Ltd
39 Milton Park
Abingdon
Oxon OX14 4TD
Tel: 0800 502030

Pressure Groups and Charities

To find out more about what is happening within the prison service, contact:
Howard League for Penal Reform
708 Holloway Rd
London N19 3NL
Tel: 0171 281 7722

Prison Reform Trust
15 Northburgh St
London EC1V 0JR
Tel: 0171 251 5070

List of references

Alderson, J. (1979) *Policing Freedom*, Plymouth: Macdonald and Evans.

Annual Report of HM Chief Inspector of Prisons. (1996–7) London: The Stationery Office.

Ashworth, A. (1993) 'Victim Impact Statements and Sentencing', *Criminal Law Review*, pp. 498–509.

Ashworth, A. (1997) *Factsheet: Race and Criminal Justice*, No.1, London: Institute for the Study and Treatment of Delinquency.

Audit Commission (1993) *Helping with Enquiries: Tackling Crime Effectively*, London: Audit Commission.

Audit Commission (1996) *Misspent Youth*, London: Audit Commission.

Audit Commission (1998a) *Misspent Youth '98: The Challenge for Youth Justice*, London: Audit Commission.

Audit Commission (1998b) *Local Authority Performance Indicators 1996/7 – Police Services*, London: Audit Commission.

Banton, M. (1973) 'Law Enforcement and Social Control' in Aubert, V. (ed.) *The Sociology of Law*, Harmondsworth: Penguin.

Barclay, G. (1995) *The Criminal Justice System in England and Wales*. London: Home Office, 3rd edition.

Bean, P., Bingley, W., Bynoe, I., Faulkner, A., Rassaby, E., and Rogers, A. (1991) *Out of Harm's Way*, London: MIND.

Blackstone, T. (1990) *Prisons and Penal Reform*. London: Chatto and Windus.

Bright, J. (1998) 'Preventing Youth Crime', *Criminal Justice Matters*, No. 33, Autumn, pp. 15–17.

Brown, D. (1997) *PACE Ten Years On: A Review of Research*, Home Office Research Findings No. 49, London.

Brown, J. (1997) 'Equal Opportunities and the Police in England and Wales: Past, Present and Future Possibilities' in Francis, P., Davies, P. and Jupp, V. (eds) *Policing Futures. The Police, Law Enforcement and the Twenty–First Century*, Basingstoke: Macmillan.

Brownlee, I. (1998) *Community Punishment. A Critical Introduction*, London: Longman.

Bucke, T. (1997) *Ethnicity and Contacts with the Police: Latest Findings from the British Crime Survey*, Home Office Research Findings No. 59, London.

Cain, M. (1973) 'On the Beat: Interactions and Relations in Rural and Urban Police Forces' in Cohen, S. (ed.) *Images of Deviance*, Harmondsworth: Penguin , pp. 62–97.

Commission for Racial Equality (1992) *A Question of Judgement: Race and Sentencing*, London: CRE.

Croall, H. (1998) *Crime and Society in Britain*, London: Longman.

Davies, M., Croall, H. and Tyrer, J. (1995) *Criminal Justice. An Introduction to the Criminal Justice System in England and Wales*, London: Longman.

Davies, M., Croall, H. and Tyrer, J. (1998) *Criminal Justice. An Introduction to the Criminal Justice System in England and Wales*, London: Longman, 2nd edition.

Dennis, N. (1998) 'Editor's Introduction' in Bratton, W., Dennis, N. (ed.), Griffiths, W., Mallon, R., Orr, J. and Pollard, C., *Zero Tolerance. Policing a Free Society*, London: Institute of Economic Affairs, London, 2nd edition, pp. 1–28.

Dennis, N. and Mallon, R. (1998) 'Confident Policing in Hartlepool' in Bratton, W., Dennis, N. (ed.), Griffiths, W., Mallon, R., Orr, J. and Pollard, C., *Zero Tolerance. Policing a Free Society*, London: Institute of Economic Affairs, 2nd edition, pp. 62–87.

Dunbar, I. and Langdon, A. (1998) *Tough Justice. Sentencing and Penal Policies in the 1990s*, London: Blackstone Press.

Edgar, K. and O'Donnell, I. (1998) *Mandatory Drug Testing in Prisons – An Evaluation*, Home Office Research Findings, No. 75, London.

Fielding, N. (1995) *Community Policing*, Oxford: Clarendon Press.

Fionda, J. (1996) *Juvenile Justice in England and Wales*, London: Institute for the Study and Treatment of Delinquency.

Flynn, N. (1998) *Introduction to Prisons and Imprisonment*, Winchester: Waterside Press.

Gibson, B. and Cavadino, P. (1995) *Introduction to the Criminal Justice Process*, Winchester: Waterside Press.

Gilling, D. (1996) 'Policing, Crime Prevention and Partnerships' in Leishman, F., Loveday, B. and Savage, S. (eds) *Core Issues in Policing*, London: Longman, pp. 101–113.

Graham, J. (1998) *Fast-Tracking of Persistent Young Offenders*, Home Office, Research Findings No. 74, London.

Grounds, A. (1992) 'Mental Health Problems' in Stockdale, E. and Casale, S. (eds) *Criminal Justice under Stress*, London: Blackstone Press, pp. 286–99.

Hagell, A. and Newburn, T. (1994) *Persistent Young Offenders*, London: Policy Studies Institute.

Harding, C. and Koffman, L. (1995) *Sentencing and the Penal System*, London: Sweet and Maxwell, 2nd edition.

Hedderman, C and Hough, M. (1994) *Does the Criminal Justice System Treat Men and Women Differently?*, Home Office, Research Findings No. 10, London.

Holdway, S. (1977) 'Changes in Urban Policing', *British Journal of Sociology*, Vol. 28, No. 2, June, pp. 119–37.

Holdaway, S. (1984) *Inside the British Police. A Force at Work*, Oxford: Basil Blackwell.

Holdaway, S. (1996) *The Racialisation of British Policing*, London: Macmillan.

Home Office (1983) *Community and Race Relations Training for the Police*, Report of the Police Training Council Working Party, London.

Home Office (1984) *Tougher Regimes in Detention Centres*, Prison Department, Home Office, HMSO.

Home Office (1989) *The 1988 British Crime Survey*, Home Office Research Study 111, London

Home Office (1995) *Young People and Crime*, Home Office Research Study 145, London.

Home Office (1996a) *An Evaluation of the Introduction and Operation of the Youth Court*, Home Office Research Study 152, London.

Home Office (1996b) *Protecting the Public: The Government's Strategy on Crime in England and Wales*, Cm 3190, London: HMSO.

Home Office (1997a) *Notifiable Offences. England and Wales, 1996*, Home Office Statistical Bulletin, London.

Home Office (1997b) *Reconvictions of Prisoners discharged from Prison in 1993, England and Wales*, Home Office Statistical Bulletin, London.

Home Office (1997c) *Reconvictions for those commencing Community Penalties in 1993, England and Wales*, Home Office Statistical Bulletin, London.

Home Office (1997d) *Race and the Criminal Justice System. A Home Office Publication under section 95 of the Criminal Justice Act 1991*, London: Criminal Policy Strategy Unit.

Home Office (1997e) *Ethnic Monitoring in Police Forces: A Beginning*, Home Office Research Study 173, London.

Home Office (1998a) *Reducing Offending. An Assessment of Research Evidence on Ways of Dealing with Offending Behaviour.* Home Office Research Study 187, London.

Home Office (1998b) *Sentencing Practice: An Examination of Decisions in Magistrates' Courts and the Crown Courts in the mid-1990s.* Home Office Research Study 180, London.

Home Office (1998c) *The Prison Population in 1997*, Home Office Statistical Bulletin, London.

Home Office (1998d) *Cautions, Court Proceedings and Sentencing. England and Wales 1997*, Home Office Statistical Bulletin, London.

Home Office (1998e) *Statistics on Race and the Criminal Justice System. A Home Office Publication under section 95 of the Criminal Justice Act 1991*, London.

Hood, R. (1992) *Race and Sentencing: A Study in the Crown Court*, Oxford: Oxford University Press.

Hough, M. and Tilley, N. (1998) *Auditing Crime and Disorder: Guidance for Local Partnerships*, Home Office, Police Research Group, Crime Detection and Prevention Series, Paper 91, London.

Howard League for Penal Reform (1997a) *A Day in the Life of a Prisoner*, Fact Sheet No. 9, London.

Howard League for Penal Reform (1997b) *Useful Facts*, Fact Sheet No. 30, London.

Howard League for Penal Reform (1997c) *Suicide and Self Injury in Prison*, Fact Sheet No. 19, London.

Howard League for Penal Reform (1997d) *Women in Prison*, Fact Sheet No. 7, London.

Howard League for Penal Reform (1997e) *The Use of Imprisonment for Girls*, Fact Sheet No. 16, London.

Howard League for Penal Reform (1997f) *Secure Training Centres: Repeating Past Failures*, London.

Howard League for Penal Reform (1997g) *Lost Inside – The Imprisonment of Teenage Girls*, London.

Howard League for Penal Reform (1998a) *Sentenced to Fail – Out of Sight, Out of Mind. Compounding the Problems of Children in Prison*, London.

Howard League for Penal Reform (1998b) *Howard League Magazine*, Vol. 16, No. 3, August, London.

James, A. and Raine, J. (1998) *The New Politics of Criminal Justice*, London: Longman.

Jordan, P. (1998) 'Effective Policing Strategies for reducing Crime' in Goldblatt, P. and Lewis, C. (eds) *Reducing Offending: An Assessment of Research Evidence on Ways of dealing with Offending Behaviour*, Home Office Research Study No. 187, London, pp. 63–81.

Kershaw, C. (1997) *Reconvictions of those commencing Community Penalties in 1993, England and Wales*, Home Office Statistical Bulletin, London.

Leigh, A., Read, T. and Tilley, N. (1998) *Brit Pop II: Problem-Oriented Policing in Practice*, Home Office, Policing and Reducing Crime Unit, Police Research Series, Paper 93, London.

Macpherson, W. (1999) *The Stephen Lawrence Inquiry*, CM 4262–I, London: The Stationery Office.

Manwaring-White, S. (1983) *The Policing Revolution. Police Technology, Democracy and Liberty in Britain*, Brighton: Harvester Press.

May, C. (1997) *Magistrates' Views of the Probation Service*, Home Office Research Findings No. 48, London.

McConville, M. and Shepherd, D. (1992) *Watching Police, Watching Communities*, London: Routledge.

McIlroy, J. (1985) 'Police and Pickets: The Law against Miners', in Beynon, J. (ed.) *Digging Deeper*, London: Verso, pp. 101–22.

Mirrlees-Black, C. and Budd, T. (1997) *Policing and the Public: Findings from the 1996 British Crime Survey*, Home Office Research Findings No. 60, London.

Mirrlees-Black, C. and Allen, J. (1998) *Concern about Crime: Findings from the 1998 British Crime Survey*, Home Office Research Findings No.83, London.

Mirrlees-Black, C., Budd, T., Partridge, S. and Mayhew, P. (1998) *The 1998 British Crime Survey. England and Wales*, Home Office Statistical Bulletin, London.

Morgan, R. and Newburn, T. (1997) *The Future of Policing*, Oxford: Oxford University Press.

Mortimer, E. and May, C. (1998) *Electronic Monitoring of Curfew Orders. The Second Year of the Trials*, Home Office Research Findings No. 66, London.

Murphy, G. (1986) *Special Care. Improving the Police Response to the Mentally Disabled*, Police Executive Research Forum, Washington, DC.

NACRO (1991) *Race and Criminal Justice*, Briefing paper, No. 77, London.

NACRO (1997a) *A New Three Rs for Young Offenders. Towards a New Strategy for Children who offend*, London: NACRO Young Offenders Committee.

NACRO (1997b) *Criminal Justice Digest*, No. 94, October, London.

NACRO (1998a) *Criminal Justice Digest*, No. 95, January, London.

NACRO (1998b) *Criminal Justice Digest*, No. 97, July, London.

NACRO (1998c) *Safer Society*, No. 1, October, London.

NCCL (1984) *Civil Liberties and the Miners' Dispute*, London: National Council for Civil Liberties.

Newburn, T. (1995) *Crime and Criminal Justice Policy*. London: Longman.

O'Donnell, I. and Edgar, K. (1996) *Victimisation in Prisons*, Home Office Research Findings, No. 37, London.

Oxford K. (1984) 'Policing by Consent' in Benyon, J. (ed.) *Scarman and After*, Oxford: Pergamon Press, pp. 114–24.

Penal Affairs Consortium (1995) *The Electronic Monitoring of Offenders*, London.

Penal Affairs Consortium (1996) *Race and Criminal Justice*, London.

Penal Affairs Consortium (1998) *An Unsuitable Place for Treatment*, London.

Percy, A. (1998) *Ethnicity and Victimization: Findings from the 1996 British Crime Survey*, Home Office Statistical Bulletin, London.

Plotnikoff, J. and Woolfson, R. (1998) *Witness Care in Magistrates' Courts and the Youth Court*, Home Office, Research Findings No. 68, London.

Pollard, C. (1998) 'Zero Tolerance: Short-term Fix, Long-term Liability?' in Bratton, W., Dennis, N. (ed.), Griffiths, W., Mallon, R., Orr, J. and Pollard, C., *Zero Tolerance. Policing a Free Society*, London: Institute of Economic Affairs, 2nd edition, pp. 44–61.

Povey, D. and Prime, J. (1998) *Notifiable Offences. England and Wales, April 1997 to March 1998*, Home Office Statistical Bulletin, London.

Prime, J., Taylor, P. and Waters-Fuller, J. (1998) *Police Service Personnel. England and Wales, as at 31 March 1998*, Home Office Statistical Bulletin, London.

Prison Reform Trust (1997) *Sentencing: A Geographical Lottery*, Briefing Paper, London.

Prison Service (1997a) *Audit of Prison Service Resources*, London: HM Prison Service.

Prison Service (1997b) *Annual Report and Accounts, April 1996–March 1997*, London: HM Prison Service.

Punch, M. (1979) 'The Secret Social Service' in Holdaway, S. (ed.) *The British Police*, London: Edward Arnold.

Reiner, R. (1985) *The Politics of the Police*, Brighton: Wheatsheaf.

Scarman, Lord (1981) *The Brixton Disorders. 10–12 April 1981*, Home Office, Cmnd 8427, London: HMSO.

Scraton, P. (1985) *The State of the Police*, London: Pluto Press.

Sheriff, P. (1998) *Summary Probation Statistics. England and Wales 1997*, Home Office Statistical Bulletin, London.

Smith, D. and Gray, J. (1985) *Police and People in London. The PSI Report*, Aldershot: Gower.

Southgate, P. and Crisp, D. (1992) *Public Satisfaction with Police Services*, Home Office, Research and Planning Unit Paper No. 73, London: HMSO.

Stead, P. J. (1985) *The Police of Britain*, New York: Macmillan Publishing Company.

Stephens, M. (1988) *Policing: The Critical Issues*, Hemel Hempstead: Harvester Wheatsheaf.

Stephens, M. (1994a) 'Care and Control: The Future of British Policing', *Policing and Society*, Vol. 4, pp. 237–51.

Stephens, M. (1994b) 'Can the Police establish a Caring Role in Community Mental Health Procedures?', *Care in Place*, Vol. 1, No. 1, pp. 65–76.

Stephens, M. and Becker, S. (1994) *Police Force, Police Service. Care and Control in Britain*. London: Macmillan.

Stockdale, E. and Casale, S. (eds) (1992) *Criminal Justice under Stress*, London: Blackstone Press.

Stockdale, J. and Gresham, P. (1998) *Tackling Street Robbery: A Comparative Evaluation of Operation Eagle Eye*, Police Research Group, Crime Detection and Prevention Series, Paper 87, London: Home Office.

Straw, J. (1998), 'How to make our prisons work', *The Independent*, 3 August.

Sugg, D. (1998) *Motor Projects in England and Wales: An Evaluation*, Home Office Research Findings No. 81, London.

Tarling, R. (1993) *Analysing Offending: Data, Models and Interpretations*, London: HMSO.

Teplin, L. (1984) 'Managing Disorder: Police Handling of the Mentally Ill' in L. Teplin (ed.) *Mental Health and Criminal Justice*, Beverley Hills: Sage, pp. 157–75.

Turner, E. and Alexandrou, B. (1997) *Neighbourhood Watch Co-ordinators*, Home Office Research Findings No. 63, London.

Vennard, J., Hedderman, C. and Sugg, D. (1997) *Changing Offenders' Attitudes and Behaviour: What Works?*, Home Office Research Findings No. 61, London.

Waddington, P. A. J. (1994) *Liberty and Order. Public Order Policing in a Capital City*, London: UCL Press.

Walker, M., Jefferson, T. and Seneviratne, M. (1989) *Ethnic Minorities, Young People and the Criminal Justice System*, London: Economic and Social Research Council.

Walklate, S. (1996) 'Equal Opportunities and the Future of Policing' in Leishman, F., Loveday, B. and Savage, S. (eds) *Core Issues in Policing*, London: Longman, pp. 191–204.

Wasik, M., Gibbons, T. and Redmayne, M. (1999) *Criminal Justice. Text and Materials*, London: Longman.

Watson, L. (1996) *Victims of Violent Crime Recorded by the Police, England and Wales, 1990–1994*, Home Office Statistical Findings, London.

White Paper (1990) *Crime, Justice and Protecting the Public*, Cm 965, London: HM Stationery Office.

White, P. (1998) *The Prison Population in 1997: A Statistical Review*, Home Office Research Findings No. 76, London.

White, P. and Powar, I. (1998) *Revised Projections of Long Term Trends in the Prison Population to 2005*, Home Office Statistical Bulletin. No. 2, London.

Willis, C. (1983) *The Use, Effectiveness and Impact of Police Stop and Search Powers*, London: Home Office Research Unit.

Wilson, D. and Ashton, J. (1998) *What Everyone in Britain should know about Crime and Punishment*, London: Blackstone Press.

Worrall, A. (1997) *Punishment in the Community. The Future of Criminal Justice*, London: Longman.

Zedner, L. (1997) 'Victims' in Maguire, M., Morgan, R. and Reiner, R. (eds) *The Oxford Handbook of Criminology*, Oxford: Clarendon Press, 2nd edition.

Index